90 0808371 2

D1756860

Cluster and Classification Techniques for the Biosciences

Recent advances in experimental methods have resulted in the generation of enormous volumes of data across the life sciences. Hence clustering and classification techniques that were once predominantly the domain of ecologists are now being used more widely. This book provides an overview of these important data analysis methods, from long-established statistical methods to more recent machine learning techniques. It aims to provide a framework that will enable the reader to recognise the assumptions and constraints that are implicit in all such techniques. Important generic issues are discussed first and then the major families of algorithms are described. Throughout the focus is on explanation and understanding and readers are directed to other resources that provide additional mathematical rigour when it is required. Examples taken from across the whole of biology, including bioinformatics, are provided throughout the book to illustrate the key concepts and each technique's potential.

ALAN H. FIELDING is Senior Lecturer in the Division of Biology at Manchester Metropolitan University.

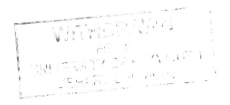

Cluster and Classification Techniques for the Biosciences

Alan H. Fielding

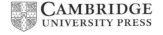

CAMBRIDGE UNIVERSITY PRESS

CAMBRIDGE UNIVERSITY PRESS
Cambridge, New York, Melbourne, Madrid, Cape Town, Singapore, São Paulo

Cambridge University Press
The Edinburgh Building, Cambridge CB2 2RU, UK

Published in the United States of America by Cambridge University Press,
New York

www.cambridge.org
Information on this title: www.cambridge.org/9780521852814

First published 2007

Printed in the United Kingdom at the University Press, Cambridge

A catalogue record for this book is available from the British Library

Library of Congress Cataloging in Publication Data

Fielding, Alan,
  Cluster and classification techniques for the biosciences / Alan H. Fielding.
     p. ; cm.
  Includes bibliographical references and index.
  ISBN-13: 978-0-521-85281-4 (hardback)
  ISBN-10: 0-521-85281-1 (hardback)
  ISBN-10: 0-521-61800-2 (pbk.)
1. Biology–Data processing. 2. Biology–Classification. 3. Cluster analysis. I. Title.
  [DNLM: 1. Cluster Analysis. 2. Biometry–methods. 3. Classification–methods. 4. Data
Interpretation, Statistical. 5. Multivariate Analysis.   WA 950 F459c 2007]
  QH324.2F537 2007
  570.285–dc22   2006027983

ISBN-13   978-0-521-85281-4   hardback
ISBN-10   0-521-85281-1   hardback

ISBN-13   978-0-521-61800-7   paperback
ISBN-10   0-521-61800-2   paperback

Dedication

This book is dedicated to the memory of Derek Ratcliffe. Derek, who was one of Britain's most important biologists, died during the writing of this book. I had the great pleasure of helping him in some very small ways with data analyses and he kindly provided a reference for my Leverhulme Fellowship award. His humility, breadth, insight and commitment are a great inspiration.

Contents

Preface

When I was originally asked to write this book I said no, several times. My reticence was a consequence of workload and not because I thought there was no need for the book. However, Katrina Halliday from Cambridge University Press persisted and eventually I gave in. However, I can only blame myself for any errors or omissions in the text.

Katrina asked me because of my editorship of an earlier machine learning book and favourable comments about some of my web material, in particular a postgraduate multivariate statistics unit. My interest in multivariate statistics arose from my research as a conservation biologist. As part of this research I spent time trying to develop predictive species distribution models, which led to my exploration of two additional topics: machine learning methods as alternatives to statistical approaches; and how to measure the accuracy of a model's predictions.

If you are not an ecologist you may be thinking that there will be little of value for you in the book. Hopefully, the contents will alleviate these fears. My multivariate statistics unit was delivered to a diverse group of students including biomedical scientists, so I am used to looking beyond ecology and conservation. In my experience there is much to be gained by straying outside of the normal boundaries of our research. Indeed my own research into the accuracy of ecological models drew greatly on ideas from biomedical research. At a fundamental level there is a great deal of similarity between a table of species abundance across a range of sites and a table of gene expression profiles across a range of samples. The subject-specific information is obviously important in devising the questions to be answered and the interpretation of results, but it is important to be aware that someone in another discipline may already have devised a suitable approach for a similar problem. Classifiers are in use in many biological and related disciplines; unfortunately there seems to be little cross-fertilisation. Throughout the book I have attempted to draw examples from a wide range of sources including ecology and bioinformatics. I hope that readers will recognise that other disciplines may already have a solution to their problem, or at least a catalogue of the difficulties and pitfalls!

As you read this text you may notice a low equation and symbol count. While this opens the text up to some obvious criticism I feel that the additional accessibility benefits outweigh the deficiencies. I am ready, if somewhat nervous, to face the reviewers' criticisms. While there are many good printed and online resources, which provide the necessary theoretical detail, I think that there is a shortage of overview resources which attempt to provide a framework that is not clouded by too much technical detail. However, the readers are expected to have some basic understanding of statistical methods. What many biologists need, and what I hope to achieve, is support in deciding if their problem can be investigated using a clustering or classification algorithm. I hope to do this by providing general guidelines and examples drawn from across biology. Given the ephemeral nature of many web pages there are relatively few web links in the text. The main exceptions are classic 'papers' and data or software sources.

During the writing several colleagues have commented on parts of the text. I am particularly grateful to Paul Craze, Les May and Emma Shaw. My research colleagues (Paul Haworth, Phil Whitfield and David McLeod) kept me entertained and revitalised during the several research meetings that we had while I was writing this book. However, I fear they may be responsible for physiological damage!

Finally, this book could not have been written without the continuing support of my wife Sue and daughter Rosie.

1

Introduction

1.1   Background

Searching for patterns in biological data has a long history, perhaps best typified by the taxonomists who arranged species into groups based on their similarities and differences. As computer resources improved there was a growth in the scope and availability of new computational methods. Some of the first biologists to exploit these methods worked in disciplines such as vegetation ecology. Vegetation ecologists often collect species data from many quadrats and they require methods that will organise the data so that relevant structures are revealed. The increase in computer power, and the parallel growth in software, allowed analyses that were previously impractical for other than small data sets.

However, the greatest data analysis challenges are undoubtedly more recent. Advances in experimental methods have generated, and continue to generate, enormous volumes of genetic information that present significant storage, retrieval and analysis challenges see Slonim (2002) for a useful review. Simultaneously there has been a growth in non-biological commercial databases and the belief that they contain information which can be used to improve company profits. One consequence of these challenges is that there is now a wide, and increasing, variety of analysis tools that have the potential to extract important information from biological data.

The analysis tools that extract information from data can be placed into two broad and overlapping categories: cluster and classification methods. This book examines a wide range of techniques from both categories to illustrate their potential for biological research. For example, they can be used to:

1. find patterns in gene expression profiles or biodiversity survey data;
2. identify class membership from some predictor variables (e.g. type of cancer, sex of a specimen, used or unused habitat);
3. identify features that either contribute to class membership or can be used to predict class membership.

1.2   Book structure

This chapter introduces the main themes and defines some terms that are used throughout the rest of the book. Chapter 2 outlines the important roles for exploratory data analysis prior to formal clustering and classification analyses. The main part of this chapter introduces multivariate approaches, such as principal components analysis and multi-dimensional scaling, which can be used to reduce the dimensionality of a dataset. They also have a role in the clustering of data. Chapter 3 examines different approaches to the clustering of biological data. The next three chapters, 4 to 6, are concerned with classification, i.e. placing objects into known classes. Chapter 4 outlines some issues that are common to all classification methods while Chapters 5 and 6 examine traditional statistical approaches and a variety of more recent, 'non-statistical', methods. Chapter 7 is related to the classification chapters because it examines the difficulties of assessing the accuracy of a set of predictions.

Although the methods covered in the book are capable of analysing very large data sets, only small data sets are used for illustrative purposes. Most data sets are described and listed in separate appendices. Others are freely available from a range of online sources.

1.3   Classification

Classification is the placing of objects into predefined groups, the archetypal biological example being identifying a biological specimen (assigning a species name). This type of process is also called 'pattern recognition', which is defined by Wikipedia (2005) as 'a field within the area of machine learning and can be defined as "the act of taking in raw data and taking an action based on the category of the data. As such, it is a collection of methods for supervised learning" '. The terms 'machine learning' and 'supervised learning' are defined in Section 1.6. However, classification is used here in a more general sense to include an element of prediction. For example, do we expect to find a species in a particular habitat (species distribution modelling), or given a particular genetic profile do we expect an individual to belong to a disease-free or disease-prone class?

Despite this increased breadth for the definition, it excludes the type of statistical predictions generated by, for example, a linear regression. Techniques such as linear regression predict a continuous, quantitative value, e.g. the expected yield of a crop given a certain fertiliser application. In this text prediction is applied almost exclusively to the identification of class membership, a categorical variable. Techniques, such as logistic regression and artificial neural networks, which produce a real-valued output (often between 0 and 1) that is subsequently split into discrete categories by the application of some threshold value, are included. Throughout this text the term classifier is used to describe a general predictive technique which allocates cases to a small number of predefined classes.

1.4   Clustering

Clustering is related to classification. Both techniques place objects into groups or classes. The important difference is that the classes are not predefined in a cluster analysis. Instead objects are placed into 'natural' groups. The term natural is a little misleading since the groupings are almost entirely dependent on the protocols that were established before starting the clustering. Clustering and classification approaches differ in the type of 'learning' method used. Classification methods use supervised methods while clustering algorithms are unsupervised (see Section 1.6). It is also important to realise that there is no concept of accuracy for an unsupervised classification, the only way of judging the outcome is by its 'usefulness'. For example, is the classification 'fit for purpose'? If it is not then one should rethink the analysis.

There is some unfortunate confusion in the use of terms. For example, Gordon's (1981, 1999) excellent books have 'Classification' as the title, but they are entirely concerned with clustering of data. In this text classification is restricted to supervised classification methods.

1.5   Structures in data

1.5.1   *Structure in tables*

A common starting point for all clustering and classification algorithms is a table in which rows represent cases (objects) and columns are the variables. Once data are in this format their original source, for example microarrays, quadrats, etc., is largely irrelevant. The hope is that we can find some structure (signals) in these data that enable us to test or develop biological hypotheses. If the data contain one or more signals there will be some structure within the table. The role of a cluster or classification analysis is to recognise the structure.

In the simplest case this structure may be masked by something as simple as the current row and column ordering. Table 1.1 is a simple example in which there is no obvious structure.

A clear structure becomes apparent once the rows and columns are reordered (Table 1.2). Unfortunately, analysing real data is rarely that simple. Although few clustering and classification algorithms explicitly re-order the table, they will generate information which reveals the presence of some structure. This topic is covered again in Chapter 2.

1.5.2   *Graphical identification of structure*

Looking for structures in data tables is only feasible when the table dimensions are relatively small. As tables become larger graphical summaries become more useful. Principal components analysis (Chapter 2) is a commonly used method that can reveal structures in interval data. As an example the data from Table 1.1 were subjected to an analysis. At the end of the analysis each case has a score for two new variables, PC1 and PC2. If these scores are plotted against each other it is obvious that there is some structure to these data (Figure 1.1). Note that the points are arranged in the same order as the re-ordered table (Table 1.2). No further explanation or interpretation is presented here but it is obvious that this approach can reveal structures in data tables.

Table 1.1. *A simple dataset with ten cases (1–10) and nine variables (a–i)*

Case	a	b	c	d	e	f	g	h	i
1	2	0	1	4	0	5	3	0	0
2	2	4	3	0	5	0	1	4	3
3	1	3	2	0	4	0	0	5	4
4	0	1	0	0	2	0	0	3	4
5	4	4	5	2	3	1	3	2	1
6	3	5	4	1	4	0	2	3	2
7	5	3	4	3	2	2	4	1	0
8	3	1	2	5	0	4	4	0	0
9	4	2	3	4	1	3	5	0	0
10	0	2	1	0	3	0	0	4	5

Table 1.2. *The dataset from Table 1.1 with re-ordered rows and columns. Zeros have been removed to highlight the structure*

Case	f	d	g	a	c	b	e	h	i
1	5	4	3	2	1				
8	4	5	4	3	2	1			
9	3	4	5	4	3	2	1		
7	2	3	4	5	4	3	2	1	
5	1	2	3	4	5	4	3	2	1
6		1	2	3	4	5	4	3	2
2			1	2	3	4	5	4	3
3				1	2	3	4	5	4
10					1	2	3	4	5
4						1	2	3	4

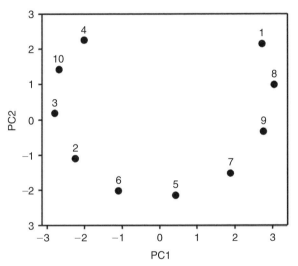

Figure 1.1 Principal component score plot for the data from Table 1.1. Points are labelled with the case numbers.

1.6   Glossary

The fields of clustering and classification are awash with terms and acronyms that may be unfamiliar. This is not helped by redundancy and overlap in their use. For example, some methods have more than one name while the same term may be used for completely different methods. The following is a short glossary of some of the more important terms that appear throughout the book.

1.6.1   *Algorithm*

An algorithm is a finite set of unambiguous instructions that describe each step needed to accomplish a task. Normally, the term refers to the design of a computer program. An algorithm differs from an heuristic (chance-based) approach because, given some initial state, it always produces the same result. For example, given a shuffled deck of playing cards, the following simple algorithm will always produce a pile of red cards on the left and a pile of black cards on the right. The order of the cards in each pile will be random.

> Repeat
>   Turn over the top card.
>   If it is red place it to the left of the shuffled deck.
>   If it is black place it to the right of the shuffled deck.
> Until no cards remain

1.6.2   *Bias*

Bias is the difference between the estimate of a value and its true value. A low bias is a desirable property for all classifiers. Unfortunately this may be difficult to achieve given the need to trade off bias against variance. Bias and variance are two parameters that feature significantly in the evaluation of classifier performance.

1.6.3   *Deviance*

The deviance is a measure of the variation unexplained by a model and is, therefore, a guide to the fit of data to a statistical model. It is calculated as twice the log-likelihood of the best model minus the log-likelihood of the current model. The best model is generally a saturated model (see maximum likelihood estimation).

1.6.4   *Learning*

Supervised learning

The use of the term 'learning' is potentially fraught with problems when biologists are involved (see Stevens-Wood (1999) for a review of 'real learning' within the context of machine learning algorithms). However, learning, as applied to classifier development, refers to the gradual reduction in error as training cases are presented to the classifier. This is an iterative process with the amount of error reducing through each iteration as the classifier 'learns' from the training cases. Supervised learning applies to algorithms in which a 'teacher' continually assesses, or supervises, the classifier's performance during training by marking predictions as correct or incorrect. Naturally, this assumes that each case has a valid class label. Learning in this sense relates to the way in which a set of parameter values are adjusted to improve the classifier's performance. However, as Hand (1997, p. 41) points out 'one may ask what is the difference between "learning" and the less glamorous sounding "recursive parameter estimation"'. The answer is, of course, none!

Unsupervised learning

In unsupervised learning there is no teacher and the classifier is left to find its own classes (also known as groups or clusters). The assumption is that there are 'natural' classes that the classifier will identify, albeit with some post-classification processing by the user. A typical example would be finding habitat classes in a satellite image or patterns in gene expression levels that may represent a particular cell state. The biggest gains from an unsupervised classification are likely in knowledge-poor environments, particularly when there are large amounts of unlabelled data. In these situations unsupervised learning can be used as a type of exploratory data analysis (Chapter 2) which may provide some evidence about the underlying structures in the data. As such it should be viewed as a means of generating, rather than testing, hypotheses.

Machine learning

Machine learning (ML) is a subset of artificial intelligence (AI) and incorporates a large number of statistical ideas and methods and uses algorithms that 'learn' from data. Learning is based around finding the relationship between a set of features and class labels in a set of training examples (supervised learning).

Induction and deduction are two types of reasoning. Induction, the leap from the particular to the general ('seeing the woods through the trees'), can be used to generate classification rules from examples by establishing 'cause−effect' relationships between existing facts (Giraud-Carrier and Martinez, 1995). For example, an inductive system may be able to recognise patterns in chess games without having any knowledge of the rules (Quinlan, 1983). Perhaps a similar system could recognise patterns in gene expression without understanding the rules that control them. Deduction is concerned with reasoning using existing knowledge. Thus, in the chess example it would be necessary to know the rules of chess before reasoning about the patterns. The requirement for previously acquired knowledge is one of the main differences between deduction and induction. Because deduction can be used to predict the consequences of events or to determine the prerequisite conditions for an observed event (Giraud-Carrier and Martinez, 1995) it is at the heart of most expert systems.

Although most ML systems are based on induction there are potential problems with this approach to learning. The first is that learning by induction requires many examples (a large sample size), although this may be outweighed by the necessity for little background knowledge (Dutton and Conroy, 1996). In a knowledge-poor discipline, such as ecology, this can be a major advantage. Another problem with inductive learning systems is that they are not guaranteed to be 'future-proof', they only make use of what happened in the 'past'. Consequently noisy or contradictory data may create problems. These difficulties are not restricted to ML programs; for example, it is well known that relationships modelled by a regression analysis should not be extrapolated beyond the limits of the original data. Noise does not have consistent effects on ML algorithms; for example, artificial neural networks, genetic algorithms and instance-based methods all use 'distributed' representations of the data while others, such as decision trees and logic, do not (Quinlan, 1993). This is important because distributed representations should be less susceptible to small alterations (noise); hence they have the potential to be more robust classifiers (Dutton and Conroy, 1996).

Carbonell (1990) placed ML techniques into four major paradigms: inductive learning; analytical learning; connectionist methods; and genetic methods. The first uses inductive techniques to derive a general class description from a database of labelled cases (the training or learning set). The analytical paradigm, including methods such as case-based reasoning, uses deduction and induction to learn from exemplars (which may be a single case). The last two are rather loosely based on biological concepts. The connectionist paradigm is an approximation of a real biological neural network while the final paradigm uses simulated selection and evolution to converge towards a solution.

1.6.5   Maximum likelihood estimation

The aim of maximum likelihood estimation is to find the values for parameters that maximise the probability of obtaining a particular set of data. If the parameters of, for example, a probability distribution are known it is a relatively simple task to determine the probability of obtaining a sample with particular characteristics. However, it is common to have a sample of values obtained from a population whose parameters are unknown. The sample could have come from many different probability distributions: maximum likelihood methods find the parameters that maximise the probability of drawing that sample.

The frequent references to log-likelihoods in connection with maximum likelihood estimation are a computational short-cut, rather than a theoretical necessity. This is because maximum likelihood estimates involve the multiplication of many small probabilities which, because of rounding errors, may get truncated to zero. If logarithms are used the multiplications become additions and the truncation problem is reduced. Because probabilities are less than one they have negative logarithms which become larger as the probability declines.

1.6.6   Microarray

A microarray, or microchip, is an important bioinformatics tool that generates large amounts of data that can be subsequently processed by clustering and classification methods. Typically a microarray will have several thousand, very small DNA spots arranged in a grid on glass or other solid material. Each spot has a fragment of a DNA or RNA molecule which corresponds to part of a known gene. Messenger RNA is extracted from biological samples and reverse-transcribed into cDNA, which is then amplified by a PCR. During the PCR amplification radioactive or fluorescent nucleotides are incorporated which are later used to detect the amount of hybridisation with the DNA fragments on the chip. It is assumed that the amount of cDNA for a particular gene reflects its activity (expression level) within the biological sample. After measurement and post-processing a table of expression values is obtained for each gene within each biological sample. These are the data that are subjected to the subsequent clustering and classification procedures to identify patterns that may provide biological insights. Quackenbush's (2001) review of computational analysis methods for microarray data is a good starting point to link clustering and classification algorithms to microarray data.

1.6.7   Multicollinearity

This is an important topic in regression-type analyses. Multicollinearity occurs when predictor variables are highly correlated, or one predictor is a function of two or more of the other predictors, for example $x_1 = x_2 + x_3$. Multicollinearity is a problem because it may prevent calculations from being completed or it can lead to instability in the regression coefficients. The instability is often manifested in coefficients having the 'wrong' sign. Thus, although we may expect y to increase as x increases ($b > 0$), multicollinearity can lead to a zero or negative value for b. This obviously makes interpretation very difficult.

1.6.8   Occam's razor

Put simply Occam's razor is a philosophy that says if a choice must be made between a number of options the simplest is the best. In the context of clustering and, particularly, classification analyses this tends to relate to the number of variables or other design decisions such as the number of weights in the neural network. In general simpler models should be preferred to more complex ones. However, Domingos (1999) discusses the role of Occam's razor in classification models and argues that choosing the simplest model may not always be desirable.

1.6.9   Ordination

Ordination is a term that is normally applied to a particular class of multivariate techniques when they are applied to ecological data. Generally they are geometrical projection methods that attempt to present multivariate data in fewer dimensions. Palmer's 'Ordination Methods for Ecologists' website has more details (http://ordination.okstate.edu/).

1.7   Recommended reading and other resources

1.7.1   Books

There are many good books that include the topics covered in this book. However, most of them have a restricted coverage, although this is usually combined with a greater depth. I have avoided the temptation to recommend subject-specific texts because the terminology and examples often obscure their explanations for readers from other disciplines. For example, Legendre and Legendre (1998) is an excellent, comprehensive book but non-ecologists may find some of the detail unhelpful. Dudoit and Fridlyand (2003) surveyed the use of microarray data in classification problems. The book by Davis (1986), which is aimed at geologists, has the clearest description of eigen values and eigen vectors that I have ever read. Unsurprisingly there are many books which fall within the machine learning and data mining spheres that may be useful. Most of these are listed in the relevant chapters but there are three that are particularly useful. First is the excellent book by Duda *et al.* (2001) which has very clear explanations for much of the theoretical background. Anyone interested in applying clustering and classification methods to their data will benefit from spending time reading this book. Second is Hand's (1997) excellent book on classification rules, which is particularly strong on assessing the performance of classifiers. The final book is Michie *et al.* (1994) which draws together the results from a series of comparative analyses. It has the added advantage of being available in a free download format.

1.7.2   Software

There are many commercial packages but often people would like to try out analyses using free software. Fortunately there are several free, but professional, packages available. The two packages listed below are general purpose, and there are many other packages that are restricted to a small number of analyses or disciplines. For example, Eisen (http://rana.lbl.gov/EisenSoftware.htm) has produced a range of clustering software for use with microarray experiments, in particular Cluster and TreeView is an integrated pair of programs for analysing and visualising the results. For example, Cluster performs a number of cluster analyses including hierarchical clustering (Chapter 3), self-organising maps (Chapter 6), k-means clustering (Chapter 3) and PCA (Chapter 2).

R (http://www.r-project.org/) is a programming and analysis environment that provides a wide variety of statistical and graphical techniques, including linear and nonlinear modelling, classical statistical tests, classification and clustering methods. The list of available packages is regularly updated and there are few statistical methods, including those only just developed, that are not available for R. There are also specialist installations aimed at particular disciplines. For example, Bioconductor (Gentleman *et al.*, 2004 and http://www.bioconductor.org/) is a set of analyses tailored to bioinformatics.

Weka (Witten and Frank, 2005) is not a single program. It is a large collection of machine learning algorithms for data mining tasks written in Java code (http://www.cs.waikato.ac.nz/ml/weka/). There is also a repository of datasets which are provided in a format readable by Weka programs.

PAST (Hammer *et al.*, 2001) is a compact, free multivariate analysis program which can be downloaded (for Windows) from http://folk.uio.no/ohammer/past/. Despite its primary focus as a tool for palaeontological data analysis it is very useful for other disciplines and includes routines for partitioning and hierarchical cluster analyses, Principal Components and Coordinates Analysis, Non-metric Multidimensional Scaling, Detrended Correspondence Analysis, Canonical Correspondence Analysis plus many other more specialised routines. It is a very good starting point to explore a range of methods, particularly if large data sets are avoided.

2

Exploratory data analysis

2.1   Background

It is important to understand and, if necessary, process the data before beginning any cluster or classification analysis exercises. The aim of these preliminary analyses is to check the integrity of the data and to learn something about their distributional qualities. The methods used to achieve these aims come under the general heading of exploratory data analysis or EDA. One of the greatest pioneers of EDA methods was J. W. Tukey. He defined EDA as an attitude and flexibility (Tukey, 1986). It is well worth reading Brillinger's (2002) short biography of Tukey to get a better understanding of why he held these views so strongly. If one wants to find out more about EDA methods a good, comprehensive, starting point is the online NIST Engineering Statistics handbook (NIST/SEMATECH). Do not be put off by the title, this is an excellent resource for biologists. According to the NIST handbook EDA is an approach or philosophy that employs a variety of techniques (mostly graphical) to:

- maximise insight into a data set;
- uncover underlying structure;
- extract important variables;
- detect outliers and anomalies;
- test underlying assumptions;
- develop parsimonious models; and
- determine optimal factor settings.

The first step in any EDA is to generate simple numerical or, even better, graphical summaries of the data. In addition to univariate analyses (histograms, box plots, etc.) it is generally worthwhile considering multivariate analyses.

At the simplest these will be bivariate scatter plots, possibly with different symbols indicating group membership (e.g. sex). More complex analyses use techniques that reduce the data dimensionality through linear and non-linear mapping procedures (Sections 2.6 and 2.7). Although many of these analyses are possible using standard statistical software a wider range of techniques is available in dedicated EDA software such as the public domain, multi-platform DATAPLOT (Filliben and Heckert, 2002) used in the NIST handbook. The GAP (generalised association plots) software produced by Chen (2002) and Wu and Chen (2006) is primarily aimed at bioinformatic data, but works well with other data. This software can produce some interesting graphical summaries (see Section 2.4.1).

Jeffers (1996) is an excellent example of how a range of statistical, and machine learning, methods can be used to explore a data set. Jeffers used a set of reference leaf measurements obtained from trees in the *Ulmus* (elm) genus. Wren *et al.* (2005) emphasise the increasing need for EDA within the broad context of genomic research. They present a case for exploring data through the increasing number of online databases. They suggest that such exploratory analyses, or data mining as it is known in the commercial world, is based on a premise that there are answers to questions that we have not thought of yet. Consequently the data drive the generation of hypotheses, rather than the reverse. They also suggest that data mining of these databases can be achieved using EDA methods to explore the possibility of relationships when there is no a priori expectation as to their nature. These explorations become more important because the rate of growth, and volumes of data, mean that more open-ended 'data-driven' questions can be asked. It is, however, important to recognise that some people view approaches such as data mining with considerable scepticism (see Section 2.9). Bo (2000) is a nice, downloadable review of knowledge discovery methods that also includes material covered in some of the later chapters.

2.2   Dimensionality

The dimensionality of a data set is the number of cases from which the data were recorded (n) and the number of parameters measured or recorded (p). For example, if 5 variables are recorded from 100 cases the dimensions of the data are 100 by 5.

In all clustering and classification algorithms it is desirable to have $n \gg p$. This is a particular problem for many microarray experiments in which there are likely to be a very large number of genes (p) relative to the number of samples (such as tumour samples). Consequently, an important role for EDA is reducing the dimensionality, particularly for p. This reduction is desirable for many reasons. For example, graphical summaries are important in EDA but it becomes very difficult to visualise data with more than three dimensions unless techniques such as principal components analysis (PCA) are used to reduce the dimensions to something more manageable. It may also be desirable because it enables recognition of variables that are unrelated to the problem. These variables may make the clustering and classification less successful because they add noise to the patterns, making them harder to detect.

The main aim of any dimension reduction algorithm is to map the original data onto a lower dimensional space, but with a minimum loss of information. This topic is considered in more detail in the sections dealing with variance- and distance-based projection methods (Sections 2.5 and 2.6) and cluster analysis (Chapter 3). In addition, reducing the dimensionality also reduces subsequent computational time, by a factor that depends on the algorithm.

Some methods, for example PCA, can also remove potential problems arising from correlated variables. The problem of correlated predictors is known as multicollinearity and it is a particular concern when stepwise variable selection routines are used to optimise a model. The sign, magnitude and significance of model coefficients can all be affected by inter-predictor correlations.

Fodor (2002) is a comprehensive survey of dimension reduction techniques that was written for the American Department of Energy.

2.3   Goodness of fit testing

Because statistical model-based analyses typically make strong assumptions about the distributional characteristics of data it is important to verify that the data are suitable. One way of verifying data is via a goodness of fit test. These are concerned with determining how well empirical data (i.e. experimental or observational data) match the characteristics expected from some theoretical probability distribution. There are three stages to goodness of fit testing.

1. Select some theoretical distribution(s) to which you expect the empirical data to conform. Usually this is based on prior knowledge and the data type. For example, if the data are counts of rare events it is possible that the data were obtained from a Poisson distribution.

2. Decide on the parameter values that characterise a particular version of the general theoretical distribution. For example, what values of n and p should be used for a candidate binomial distribution, what mean and standard deviation characterise a normal distribution? Several methods are available, including ordinary least squares (OLS) and weighted least

squares (WLS) and maximum likelihood techniques. Each has their own advantages and disadvantages.

3. Compare the empirical data with the expected (theoretical) values using a statistical test and/or a graphical method. In general goodness of fit is measured by subtracting observed values from expected values (those predicted by the model with fitted parameter values). Thus, a residual is calculated, which will be close to zero if the fit is good. In some circumstances entire probability distributions must be compared using methods that compare the empirical distribution functions (EDFs) of the test data to the cumulative distribution function (CDF) of a specified candidate parametric probability distribution.

More detailed treatment of these approaches can be found in two down-loadable resources. Chapter 2 of the online USGS *Statistical Methods in Water Resources* (Helsel and Hirsch, 2005) or Chapter 1 of the *Options for Development of Parametric Probability Distributions for Exposure Factors* online book from the US Environmental Protection Agency (Myers *et al.*, 2000).

2.4   Graphical methods

2.4.1   *Background*

There are two important pioneers in the use of graphics to understand data. The first was Tukey who invented methods such as the box and whisker plot. It is important to understand that he viewed these graphical summaries as important guides that should be used in an iterative process to assist in the development and refinement of hypotheses which would be tested later. The second, and perhaps less well known, pioneer was Jacques Bertin. He developed theories that he called the semiology of graphics which are set out in his book that predates all computer graphics (Bertin, 1967). Bertin was concerned with combining design and science to create graphics that treat data so that they convey information. Central to many of Bertin's ideas is the concept of the orderable matrix in which data are reduced to a series of row and column summaries that can then be reordered to highlight important data structures and exceptions (see Table 1.1). Good examples of this approach, although with different names, are the bi-directional cluster plots that are used to visual gene expression profiles (e.g. Chen's (2002) generalised association plots), while Friendly (2002) described a graphical summary method for depicting the patterns of correlations among variables that uses various renderings to depict the signs and magnitudes of correlation coefficients in a table that has had its rows and columns reordered. Similarly, archaeologists use a method called seriation which reorders a table so that presence values are concentrated along the table's diagonal. The earlier work of Tukey and Bertin has been greatly extended by the opportunities afforded by high-speed computers and enhanced graphical capabilities (e.g. Tufte, 1997).

2.5   Variance-based data projections

2.5.1   *Background*

When multivariate interval data are collected it is common to find some correlated variables. One implication of these correlations is that there will be redundancy in the information provided by the variables. In the extreme case of two perfectly correlated variables (x and y) one is redundant. Knowing the value of x leaves y with no freedom and vice versa. PCA and the closely related factor analysis exploit the redundancy in multivariate data by picking out patterns (relationships) in the variables and reducing the dimensionality of a data set without a significant loss of information.

PCA differs from distance-based dimension reduction techniques such as multidimensional scaling because PCA attempts to maximise the variance retained by new variables while they attempt to maintain the distances between cases.

Note that the method is principal ('first in rank or importance', Concise Oxford Dictionary) not principle ('a fundamental truth or law as the basis of reasoning or action', Concise Oxford Dictionary) components analysis.

2.5.2   *PCA*

Outline

PCA is a technique that transforms an original set of variables (strictly continuous variables) into derived variables that are orthogonal (uncorrelated) and account for decreasing amounts of the total variance in the original set. These derived variables, or components, are linear combinations of the original variables. Each variable makes a contribution to a component that is determined by the magnitude of its loading. The pattern of the loadings can be used to interpret the 'meaning' of the components. The first component usually conveys information about the relative 'sizes' of the cases and more interesting information is likely to be held in the subsequent components. In many analyses most of the information from the original variables will be retained in the first few components. Because these have a lower dimension it is usually possible to examine graphical summaries that may reveal some of the structures within the data. Because interpretation of the components is based on patterns in the loadings it is sometimes useful to rotate the new components in such a way that the loadings change into a more interpretable pattern.

Many statistical texts explain that multivariate normality is an important assumption for a valid PCA. However, since the analysis is not used to test statistical hypotheses any violations of the assumptions will only impact on the usefulness of the analysis as a guide to the identification of structure. Although there is an assumption that the original variables are continuous, it is generally acceptable to include some discrete variables while categorical variables can be recoded as a series of binary variables. Ultimately the success of the analysis, which is mainly exploratory, should be judged by the usefulness of its interpretation.

PCA has a data pre-processing role because it can create uncorrelated predictors that are important for techniques such as multiple regression. Ben-Hur and Guyon (2003) also recommended PCA prior to clustering because they suggest that the directions with most variance are the most relevant to the clustering. Thus, PCA could be used to filter out data that had low variance resulting from similar values across all cases. However, they also suggest that the PCA should use the covariance matrix rather than the standardised correlation matrix (see below).

Matrix methods (a very brief review)

It is difficult to fully understand most multivariate methods without at least a rudimentary knowledge of matrix algebra methods. The following section very briefly outlines a number of important features that differentiate matrix methods from normal arithmetic. The reader is advised to consult other texts to obtain the necessary detail for these methods.

Matrix or linear algebra methods make use of data stored as vectors or matrices. A vector is either a row or a column of numbers, e.g. the vector [12, 34, 24] contains three numbers, these could be the x, y, z coordinates for a point in three-dimensional space. A matrix is a table of numbers or vectors (see below). For example, the matrix below is a square, symmetrical five by five matrix of the correlation coefficients for the five variables in the next analysis. It is square because it has the same number of rows and columns and it is symmetrical because the upper right triangle of values is a mirror image of those in the lower left triangle. Matrices do not have to be square or symmetrical.

1.000	0.631	0.553	−0.030	−0.399
0.631	1.000	0.895	0.246	0.032
0.553	0.895	1.000	0.167	−0.046
−0.030	0.246	0.167	1.000	0.534
−0.399	0.032	−0.046	0.534	1.000

Most normal arithmetic operations are possible on vectors and matrices, e.g. addition, subtraction, multiplication, etc. A different set of rules are applied to some of these operations compared with normal arithmetic, although addition and subtraction are easy.

For example, let matrices A and B be

$$\begin{matrix} 4 & 3 \\ 2 & 1 \end{matrix} \quad \text{and} \quad \begin{matrix} 5 & 2 \\ 4 & 8 \end{matrix}$$

Then if C = A + B, the contents of C are

$$\begin{matrix} 9 & 5 \\ 6 & 9 \end{matrix}$$

Subtraction works in a similar way. Note that matrices must have an identical structure (same number of rows and columns) for this to be possible. Multiplication is slightly more complicated; details are not given here except to say that multiplication can only occur when the number of rows in one matrix matches the number of columns in the other, and vice versa.

The following example demonstrates the power of the matrix algebra methods to deal with potentially difficult problems. Consider the following pair of simultaneous equations:

$$3x + 4y = 18$$
$$2x + 3y = 13$$

How can we find the values for the two unknowns? The first step is to rewrite the equation in matrix format as matrix A and two column vectors $\mathbf{v}$ and $\mathbf{h}$.

A		v	h
3	4	x	18
2	3	y	13

The equation can now be written as $A\mathbf{v} = \mathbf{h}$, where $\mathbf{v}$ is a vector of the unknown values.

In the same way that any number multiplied by its inverse is one, any matrix multiplied by its inverse results in the matrix equivalent of one, the unit matrix, I (all zeros except the diagonal which are all ones).

Multiply both sides of the equation by the inverse of A (A^{-1}):

$$A^{-1}A\mathbf{v} = A^{-1}.\mathbf{h}$$

but $A^{-1}A = I$, therefore $I\mathbf{v} = A^{-1}\mathbf{h}$. The unit matrix can be ignored since it is the equivalent to multiplying by one:

$$\mathbf{v} = A^{-1}\mathbf{h}$$

Therefore, if A^{-1} can be found the equation can be solved to obtain the vector $\mathbf{v}$, and hence the values of x and y ($\mathbf{v}$ is the product of A^{-1} and $\mathbf{h}$). There are standard computational methods for finding the inverse of a matrix; however these generally require the use of a computer. For completeness, $x = 2$ and $y = 3$.

There is one matrix method that has no counterpart in the mathematics that most biologists encounter as undergraduates but it is essential for many multivariate techniques. Eigen values (also known as latent roots) and their associated eigen vectors provide a summary of the data structure represented by a symmetrical matrix (such as would be obtained from correlations, covariances or distances). The eigen value provides information about the magnitude of a dimension, while its eigen vector fixes the dimension's orientation in space. There are as many eigen values as there are dimensions in the matrix and each eigen vector will have as many values as there are dimensions in the matrix.

The following examples attempt to explain the importance, and role, of eigen values and eigen vectors using a mainly graphical description. Imagine what a three-dimensional scatter plot of three uncorrelated variables (x, y and z) would look like. If the three variables share the same measurement scale the points would form a circular cloud (the shape of a tennis ball). The cloud of points (Figure 2.1) has three dimensions that are all the same length (the diameter of the cloud). A correlation matrix for these three variables would be a unit matrix with three rows and columns (each variable is perfectly correlated, $r = 1.0$, with

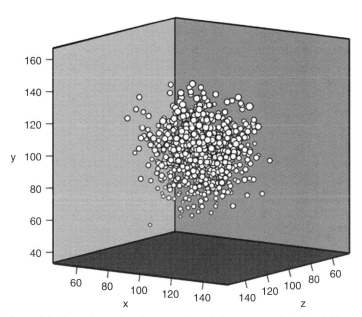

Figure 2.1 Three-dimensional scatter plot of three uncorrelated variables.

Table 2.1. *Correlation matrix for three variables and its eigen values and eigen vectors*

	Correlation matrix			Eigen values	Eigen vector 1	Eigen vector 2	Eigen vector 3
	x	y	z				
x	1.0	0.0	0.0	1.0	0.000	0.000	1.000
y	0.0	1.0	0.0	1.0	0.000	1.000	0.000
z	0.0	0.0	1.0	1.0	1.000	0.000	0.000

itself and has zero correlation with the other two). This matrix has a rather dull set of eigen values and eigen vectors (Table 2.1).

The relationship between the correlation matrix and its eigen values and vectors may become clearer if a second data set is considered. Imagine three variables that share a common correlation of 0.5 with each other. What will a scatter plot look like in three-dimensional space? It is easier to start in two dimensions. If two variables, with a shared measurement scale, are correlated the data points will be arranged along a diagonal axis with a spread that is related to the degree of correlation. If they are perfectly correlated the points will form a perfect line. As the correlation reduces there will be an increased scatter away from the diagonal, approximating to an ellipse that has two dimensions, a length and a breadth (Figure 2.2).

In the three-dimensional plot the scatter plot will be ellipsoid. One analogy is a rugby ball or American football. Like the previous tennis ball this also has three dimensions (length, width and depth) but this time they are not equal, although two (width and depth) should be very similar, unless the ball is beginning to deflate. This correlation matrix (Table 2.2 and Figure 2.3) has the eigen values of 2.0 ('length'), 0.5 ('width') and 0.5 ('depth'). There are several things to note about these values. Firstly, they sum to three, the dimensionality of the data; secondly, they describe the dimensions of the ellipsoid. The eigen vectors are coordinates in x, y, z space that define the orientation of each of its axes. There are no unique eigen vectors since any point along the appropriate axis would allow it to be positioned correctly. One of the common conventions that is used to determine the values in an eigen vector is that the sum of their squared values should be one. For example, the sum of the squared eigen vectors for the first eigen value is $-0.577^2 + -0.577^2 + -0.577^2 = 1.00$. This means that the longest axis of the ellipsoid has a length of 2.0 and passes through the origin (0,0,0) and a point with coordinates $-0.577, -0.577, -0.577$. The second axis, which is perpendicular to the first, has a length of 0.5 and passes through the origin and a point with the coordinates $0.085, -0.746, 0.660$.

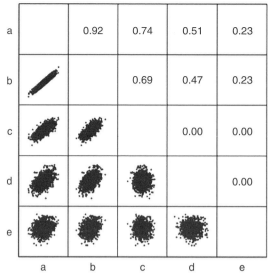

Figure 2.2 Matrix of bivariate scatter plots of five variables with decreasing correlations. Correlation coefficients are given in the upper right diagonal.

Table 2.2. *Correlation matrix for three variables and its eigen values and eigen vectors*

	Correlation matrix			Eigen values	Eigen vector 1	Eigen vector 2	Eigen vector 3
	x	*y*	*z*				
x	1.0	0.5	0.5	2.0	−0.577	0.085	−0.812
y	0.5	1.0	0.5	0.5	−0.577	−0.746	0.332
z	0.5	0.5	1.0	0.5	−0.577	0.660	0.480

The final example has a more complex correlation structure (Table 2.3). Variables x and y are almost perfectly correlated ($r = 0.9$), z has different levels of correlation with x ($r = 0.3$) and y ($r = 0.6$). Think for a moment about what this means for the effective dimensionality of the data. If all three were perfectly correlated the eigen values would be 3.0, 0.0 and 0.0 and the three-dimensional scatter plot would be a line with only a length (3.0) and no width and depth. In other words, it would only have one effective dimension. In this example, the large correlation between x and y, combined with the correlations with z, mean that the effective dimensions of these data are less than three. The eigen values are 2.23, 0.73 and 0.04. The final dimension is very small, suggesting that we could visualise the ellipsoid as a wide, but flat, two-dimensional ellipse that was almost three times longer than it was wide. In other words, the effective dimensions for these data are closer to two than three. PCA, which is based on an

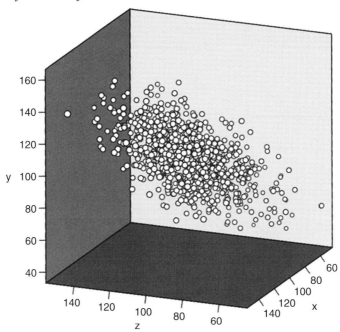

Figure 2.3 Three-dimensional scatter plot of three correlated variables ($r = 0.5$ for each pair).

eigen analysis of the correlation or covariance matrix, exploits this redundancy in data to reduce its dimensions. If any of the components has an eigen value close to zero it usually indicates that one or more variables is a linear function of the other variables and can, therefore, be constructed from their values. When this happens it means that the effective dimensionality of a data set must be less than the number of variables.

Example analysis 1

This analysis of an artificial data set (Appendix A), with a known structure (see discussion above), was carried out using Minitab (Version 14). There are 30 cases and 5 variables labelled v1 to v5. The program output is

```
Eigenvalue  2.4490   1.6497   0.5140   0.3028   0.0845
Proportion  0.490    0.330    0.103    0.061    0.017
Cumulative  0.490    0.820    0.923    0.983    1.000
```

- The first row has the eigen values of the correlation matrix.
- The second row has the proportion of variation associated with each component, e.g. for PC1 2.449/5.000 = 0.490 or 49%.

Table 2.3. *Correlation matrix for three variables and its eigen values and eigen vectors*

	Correlation matrix			Eigen values	Eigen vector 1	Eigen vector 2	Eigen vector 3
	x	y	z				
x	1.0	0.9	0.3	2.23	0.593	−0.525	0.611
y	0.9	1.0	0.6	0.73	0.658	−0.121	−0.743
z	0.3	0.6	1.0	0.04	0.464	0.842	0.273

- The third row is the cumulative variation retained by the components, e.g. 0.820 is 0.490 + 0.330.
- Most of the information (82%) is contained within the first two components.

The eigen values (2.449, 1.6497, 0.514, 0.3028 and 0.0845) sum to 5.000, the number of variables. Indeed, if the correlation matrix is analysed, their sum is always the number of variables. This is because each of the variables is standardised to a mean of zero and a variance of one. Thus, the total variance to be partitioned between the components is equal to the number of variables. Because the fifth eigen value is close to zero it indicates that at least one of the variables is a linear function of the others and the effective dimensions for these data are less than five.

Since the role of PCA is to reduce dimensionality it would be pointless to work with five components rather than the original five variables. Therefore a decision is needed on the appropriate number of components to retain. There are two guidelines in general use. The first is a scree plot of eigen values against the number of components. The appropriate number of components is indicated when the plot levels off. The second method was proposed by Kaiser and relates to standardised variables. When variables are standardised they have a variance of 1.0. This means that any component or factor, whose eigen value is less than one, retains less variance than one of the original variables. Consequently such components may be thought to convey less 'information' than the original variables and should therefore be ignored as noise. There are two aspects to this guideline that one should continually bear in mind.

1. It is only a guideline and the analysis details should be inspected to see if it should be overridden. For example, a component whose eigen value was 0.999 would not be extracted using the rule. This is clearly nonsense.

2. The rule only applies when the analysis is based on standardised variables. If the analysis is carried out on the covariance matrix of unstandardised data (whose variance may be far in excess of 1.0) then the rule should not be applied.

Tests using simulated data suggest that both methods perform quite well and generally produce similar answers. However, it is also important to use judgement, such that an interpretable solution is produced (see the stickleback analysis).

The next table has the eigen vectors, or component loadings, of the five components. Normally, because their eigen values are larger than 1.0 (the Kaiser criterion), the interpretation would be restricted to the first two components. The component loadings are used to calculate the component scores.

```
Component Loadings
Variable     PC1       PC2       PC3       PC4       PC5
   v1       -0.514    -0.260    0.477     0.631     -0.205
   v2       -0.605    -0.134    -0.228    -0.022    0.751
   v3       -0.587    -0.078    -0.381    -0.357    -0.613
   v4       -0.120    -0.652    0.667     -0.340    -0.020
   v5       0.102     -0.695    -0.361    0.598     -0.134
```

The calculation of component scores assumes that the variables have standardised scores (mean = 0, standard deviation = 1.0). The loadings, or weights, of each variable control the contributions that they make to the component scores. Because the variables share the same scale it is easy to interpret their relative importance. For example, v4 and v5 make only minor contributions to the first component, and more major contributions to the second component. The variables making the most important contribution to each component have their loading shown in bold. A 'rule of thumb' was used such that loadings >0.3 are considered important. In a real example the next stage would be an attempt to assign some name to the combination of variables associated with a component. Because component scores have a mean of zero, a negative score indicates a case with a below average score on that component, whilst a positive score indicates a case with an above average score. Obviously a case with a zero score is average.

In summary, the interpretation of these data, using PCA, is that

- The data can be represented adequately in just two dimensions.
- The first of these is associated with variables v1, v2 and v3.
- The second is associated with variables v4 and v5.

If the same data are subjected to a factor analysis the following results are obtained using Minitab (V14)

```
Unrotated Factor Loadings and Communalities
```

Variable	Factor1	Factor2	Factor3	Factor4	Factor5	Communality
V1	−0.803	0.337	0.342	0.347	−0.061	1.000
V2	**−0.947**	−0.170	−0.164	−0.009	0.219	1.000
V3	**−0.919**	−0.099	−0.274	−0.198	−0.178	1.000
V4	−0.192	**−0.837**	0.476	−0.189	−0.005	1.000
V5	0.159	**−0.894**	−0.255	**0.331**	−0.040	1.000
Variance	2.4480	1.6518	0.5110	0.3044	0.0848	5.000
% Var	0.490	0.330	0.102	0.061	0.017	1.000

```
Factor Score Coefficients
```

Variable	Factor1	Factor2	Factor3	Factor4	Factor5
V1	−0.328	0.204	0.670	1.139	−0.716
V2	−0.387	−0.103	−0.321	−0.028	2.578
V3	−0.375	−0.060	−0.536	−0.650	−2.100
V4	−0.078	0.507	0.932	−0.619	−0.059
V5	0.065	−0.541	−0.500	1.087	−0.473

The factor analysis output differs from the PCA because it has tables of factor loadings and factor score coefficients. As with the PCA eigen vectors, the factor loadings provide information about the contribution that each variable makes to a factor. The most important variables, for each factor, are again highlighted in bold. Note that the pattern is very similar to that observed in the Minitab PCA of the same data. The factor loadings are obtained from the eigen vectors by a process of 'normalisation' that involves multiplying each eigen vector by the square root (the singular value) of its eigen value. For example, for v1 component one, the PCA eigen vector is −0.513, and the square root of its eigen value (2.449) is 1.565: −0.513 × 1.565 = −0.803. If a 'pure' PCA is required the eigen vectors can be obtained from the loadings by dividing each loading by the square root of the eigen value. For example, −0.803/1.565 = −0.513. Most usefully the loadings are simple correlation coefficients between the original variables and the newly derived factors.

Example analysis 2

These data (Appendix B) relate to an experiment investigating the behaviour of male stickleback. The responses of male fish during an observation period were recorded, which included the response to a 'model' male fish. The first analysis is a simple PCA.

Eigenvalue	2.2881	1.4542	0.9791	0.8861	0.7532	0.4048	0.2344
Proportion	0.327	0.208	0.140	0.127	0.108	0.058	0.033
Cumulative	0.327	0.535	0.674	0.801	0.909	0.967	1.000

Two components have eigen values above one. Applying the Kaiser criterion would mean that only 53.5% of the variability would be retained in two components. The third component has an eigen value close to one (0.98). Retaining three components, which is supported by a scree plot, would mean that 67.4% of the variation was retained. There is also a problem with the loadings for the components (see below).

Variable	PC1	PC2	PC3	PC4	PC5	PC6	PC7
LUNGES	0.470	−0.310	−0.482	−0.076	0.181	0.055	0.639
BITES	0.459	−0.507	−0.130	0.050	0.084	0.080	−0.706
ZIGZAGS	−0.248	−0.379	0.244	−0.783	0.022	0.346	0.053
NEST	−0.435	−0.400	−0.327	−0.095	−0.114	−0.721	−0.037
SPINES	0.164	−0.465	0.622	0.324	−0.412	−0.116	0.287
DNEST	−0.422	−0.224	−0.399	0.361	−0.391	0.574	0.005
BOUT	0.335	0.275	−0.197	−0.367	−0.790	−0.089	−0.073

None of the loadings of the seven variables on the three main components are small or large, most are in the range 0.3−0.6 and hence they do little to explain the data structure. Looking at the loadings for PC1−PC3 it is not easy to say which variables are particularly associated with each component.

There is also an argument that the analysis should consider four components. The fourth component has an eigen value of 0.89, and retaining it would mean that 80% of the variation could be retained in four dimensions. Therefore, the PCA was repeated but with an option to extract four components. However, because the loadings do not change (not shown) the interpretation remains difficult.

In order to improve the interpretability the four extracted components can be subjected to a rotation. Imagine holding a novel object in your hands; in an attempt to understand it you would almost certainly turn it over and twist it around. In other words you would subject it to a rotation whose effect would be to change your view of the object, without ever changing the object itself. Rotation of a PCA solution does exactly the same thing. The aim of the rotation is to improve the interpretability of the analysis by removing, as far as possible, mid-value loadings. If loadings are either high or low the interpretation is simplified. The most widely accepted method is Varimax rotation. This is an iterative method which rotates the axes into a position such that the sum of the variances of the loadings is the maximum possible. This will occur when loadings, within each factor, are dissimilar, i.e. a mixture of high and low values. It is important to understand that Varimax rotation does not distort the original data. The rotation changes its projection onto the lower dimensions that we use to interpret the structure.

```
Rotated Factor Loadings and Communalities Varimax Rotation

Variable  Factor1   Factor2   Factor3   Factor4

LUNGES     0.921    −0.118     0.096    −0.082

BITES      0.868    −0.107    −0.331     0.000

ZIGZAGS   −0.066     0.100    −0.064     0.965

NEST      −0.011     0.784     0.092     0.395

SPINES     0.167    −0.069    −0.901     0.049

DNEST     −0.110     0.854     0.072    −0.074

BOUT       0.270    −0.535     0.406    −0.038

Variance   1.7199    1.6698    1.1137    1.1043

% Var      0.246     0.239     0.159     0.158
```

The initial (not shown) component loading matrix is identical to the four-component PCA. The important rotated loadings have been highlighted in bold. The structure is now much simpler with a more clearly delineated pattern of loadings.

1. Lunges, Bites and Bouts: may be interpreted as 'Aggression'
2. Nest, Dnest and Bouts (negative): may be interpreted as 'Nest Activity'
3. Bites, Spines and Bouts (negative): a different type of 'Aggression'
4. Zigzags and Nest: female-centred display

This is a much more successful analysis, in which the dimensionality has been reduced from seven to four and the extracted factors can be interpreted to produce a biologically reasonable interpretation.

Figure 2.4 shows the scores for the cases on the first two of the new components: 'Aggression' and 'Nest Activity'. The plot has been split into four regions, using boundaries set at zero on both axes.

1. Region A: below average on the first factor and above average on the second. Thus, these individuals did not show much aggression but spent an above average time on nest building activities.

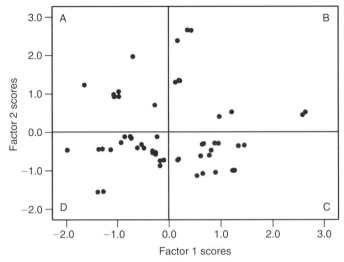

Figure 2.4 Scatter plot of factor scores for the first two principal components.

2. Region B: above average on both factors. Thus, they combine above average aggression with a lot of nest building activities. Note the lack of points along the diagonal, why? (Think about what the fish would have to do to get on the diagonal.)

3. Region C: above average on the first factor and below average on the second. These individuals did not spend much time on nest building but were above average with respect to aggression.

4. Region D: below average on both factors. These individuals did not do much!

2.5.3   Factor analysis

The similarities and differences between PCA and factor analysis (FA) create considerable confusion. This is not helped when in some software, for example SPSS, PCA is accessed via the FA menu. Both methods achieve similar aims of dimension reduction but there are important differences in the underlying models and FA can be used in an exploratory and a confirmatory role. Whereas PCA is a variance-orientated technique FA is concerned solely with correlations between variables. FA assumes that observed correlations are caused by some underlying pattern in the data resulting from the presence of a number of predetermined factors. Strictly, on the basis of some subject-specific theory, the number of factors should be known in advance. The contribution of any variable can then be split into a common component, i.e. that part which contributes to the factors, and a unique component which can be thought of as noise. The sum of the common components is called the communality. Communality values are between zero and one. A communality of zero would arise if a variable was uncorrelated with all other variables and had no shared information. The subsequent FA methodology is very similar to PCA except that the variability to be partitioned between the factors is that held in common, unique variability is excluded from the analysis. This makes sense since any unique variance cannot be contributing to a shared factor, so should be excluded.

Forcing the analysis to use as many factors as there are variables partially overcomes the differences between PCA and FA. This is demonstrated by the fact that the communalities are all 1.000, and thus all of the variability is assumed to be common and all of it will be used in the analysis (as in a PCA).

There is an argument that FA is preferable to PCA for pre-processing prior to developing a classifier or clustering. In a FA the unique variability ('noise') associated with each predictor is explicitly excluded. Consequently the data are 'smoothed', which may remove nuisance values that create complex decision boundaries.

2.6   Distance-based data projections

2.6.1   Background

In ecology the niche of a species is represented by a large number of variables (p). If the mean for each variable is used the niche becomes a single point in p-dimensional space. Similarly, the state of the genome can be represented by a single point that represents the expression values for each of p genes. A complete description of either requires that all p variables are recorded. However, once p exceeds the trivial value of three it is difficult to represent this state unless it can be mapped onto fewer dimensions. It would certainly be very difficult to compare two niches or two gene expression states visually in their original p-dimensional space. Multidimensional scaling (MDS) methods aim to provide a visual representation of the pattern of the distances between cases, but in a reduced number of dimensions. The output is a map with similar cases plotted near to each other. In this respect they are similar to PCA but there are important differences between the assumptions. In general the MDS methods have much weaker assumptions and only require a matrix of distances or similarities.

The starting point is an $n \times n$ distance matrix, Dm, which records the distance between each pair of cases measured across all p variables. This is identical to the starting point in a standard hierarchical cluster analysis (Section 3.4). Because the distance between A and B is the same as that between B and A, Dm is a symmetric matrix. A classic everyday example is the between-city distance matrix found in most road atlases. One of the main aims of these analyses is to discover if there is some underlying structure to the data, perhaps represented by clusters of cases. They also offer the opportunity to identify relationships between cases that possibly represent recognisable temporal patterns such as those found in developmental pathways or species changes following changes to ecological management practices.

Starting from the distance matrix these methods attempt to recreate the original spread of points (e.g. cities), but in reduced dimensions (typically two or three). This is achieved by finding a configuration of points, in Euclidean space, such that the distance matrix (Dc) of this new configuration is a reasonable match to Dm. Because there is no obvious solution the algorithm is iterative, using a pattern of perturbations to the trial configuration of points such that each perturbation reduces the mismatch between Dm and Dc. Note that it will rarely be possible to obtain an exact match between Dm and Dc so that some stopping criterion, such as stress, is used to identify when future improvements are too small to continue.

There are two general classes of methods that come under the general heading of metric scaling. Metric scaling methods, such as principal coordinate analysis (classic metric scaling), attempt to produce mappings such that the distances in Dc match those in Dm, albeit at a different scale. The more general non-metric scaling methods only attempt to create a mapping that retains the relative distances between cases, i.e. distances are in the correct rank order. In the same way that non-parametric statistical tests, such as the Mann Whitney U test, calculate test statistics from ranks the non-metric scaling methods use the ranks of the distances in Dm. Starting from a trial configuration an iterative algorithm is used to improve the match of the ordering of the distances.

The match between the original and trial configurations is measured using a stress or loss function. Chen and Chen (2000) developed a graphical exploratory tool to investigate how well individual cases or pairs are represented in the projected space. This is not possible using global-fitness measures such as stress. In effect their method provides tools similar to the diagnostic tools used to judge the fit of regression models.

Azuaje et al. (2005) describe how non-linear mapping techniques can be used as an exploratory tool in functional genomics. However, they do not use a standard method. Instead they tested a method devised by Chang and Lee (1973) which works with a single pair of points at each iteration, rather than adjusting the complete data set.

2.6.2   *MDS or principal coordinate analysis*

Classic MDS, which is also known as principal coordinates analysis, is a more general form of PCA. The main difference is that while PCA uses a correlation or covariance matrix, MDS can use any distance matrix. A second important difference is that, because MDS uses a distance matrix, the analysis focuses on the cases and no information is provided about the contribution of individual variables to the data structures. However, this does mean that MDS is useful when $p > n$. If a Euclidean distance matrix is used MDS and PCA produce identical projections, albeit with some possible reversal of signs, i.e. the projections may be reflections or translations. There are several example analyses in Chapter 5.

2.6.3   *Sammon mapping*

Sammon (1969) also devised a mapping algorithm which is used in biology less often than MDS or non-metric MDS. He said that his non-linear mapping algorithm aimed to 'detect and identify "structure" which may be present in a list of N L-dimensional vectors'. It is an iterative procedure that begins with an n by n distance matrix, which contains the Euclidean distances between all pairs of cases measured across all p variables. There is a second distance matrix which begins with distances calculated from random coordinates allocated to each case on a reduced number of variables (axes). A mapping error, E, is calculated by comparing the original and reduced-space distance matrices. The gradient which will minimise E is also calculated. Cases are now moved in the lower dimensional space according to the direction given by the gradient. The second distance matrix and E are recalculated. This process is continued until E drops below a specified limit. The final result is a set of coordinates for each case on the reduced number of axes, typically two or three. Sammon mapping is said to produce mappings which spread the points out more evenly than MDS or PCA, possibly because the stress function emphasises the smaller distances.

Apostol and Szpankowski (1999) used Sammon mapping to explore the relationship between protein structure and their amino acid compositions. Distances were obtained from differences in the proportions of 19 amino acids and the resulting two-dimensional projection showed that proteins belonging to the same structural classes formed distinct clusters, albeit with significant overlapping of clusters. They suggest that this overlap may explain the limited success of previous protein folding predictions based solely on amino acid composition.

2.6.4   *Non-metric multidimensional scaling (NMDS)*

The starting point is the lower triangle of a distance matrix, which need not be Euclidean. As with MDS, the aim is to transform these distances into a set of Euclidean distances in low-dimensional space. However, in NMDS the rank order of the original distances is assumed to contain the necessary information. The aim is to reproduce, as closely as possible, the rank order of the distances from the original distance matrix in the final Euclidean distance matrix. NMDS is an iterative algorithm which uses monotone regression to calculate pseudo-distances. The difference between a real and corresponding pseudo-distance is an index of how far the distance between two cases departs from the value required to preserve the original distance rank. The overall measure of how badly the distances in the current configuration fit the original data is called the stress. The raw stress score is usually normalised to range from 0 (perfect fit) to 1 (worst fit). The normalisation makes the stress score independent of the size or scale of the configuration and allows the appropriate solution dimensionality to be identified. For example, a scree plot of the stress value against different numbers of dimensions can be used to look for a break in the slope. It is also possible to use ease of interpretation as a guide to final dimensionality. For example, if there is no pattern in the projected data points it may be worth altering the number of dimensions and re-examining the plots for structure. Of course it is always possible that there is no obvious structure. If this is the case there will be no obvious break in the scree plot and plots of the data points will resemble random noise.

It is normal to have stress values greater than zero and it is important to realise that this only occurs when the solution has insufficient dimensions. Increasing the number of dimensions may reduce the stress, it can never increase it. However, since the aim is to reduce the dimensionality it is normal to accept some distortion (a stress value greater than zero). It is likely that the greatest distortions (at least proportionally) are in the smallest distances. This is because the goodness of fit measures place greater emphasis on larger dissimilarities.

2.7   Other projection methods

2.7.1   *Correspondence analysis*

A method such as PCA assumes that there are linear relationships between the derived components and the original variables. This is apparent from the role of the covariance or correlation matrix. If the relationships are non-linear a Pearson correlation coefficient, which measures the strength of linear relationships, would underestimate the strength of the non-linear relationship.

Because such non-linear relationships are quite common in biology an alternative method is frequently needed. For example, species abundance will peak at a certain temperature, while enzyme activity will show similar non-linearity with respect to pH. In fact correspondence analysis can be viewed as a weighted PCA in which Euclidean distances are replaced by chi-squared distances that are more appropriate for count data.

Correspondence analysis (or reciprocal averaging as it is also known) is a method that is quite often used in ecological analyses where non-linear relationships are common. It is less commonly used in other biological disciplines, although there are several examples where it has been used with molecular data. For example, Castresana *et al.* (2004) revealed that significant variations in evolutionary rates exist among genomic regions of human and mouse genomes, while Perrière and Thioulouse (2002) raised some concerns about the use of correspondence analysis with non-count data in codon usage studies. As with PCA, derived variables are created from the original variables but this time they maximise the correspondence between row and column counts.

There are two main algorithms used to find the solution to a correspondence analysis. The first is an iterative algorithm that gives the method its alternative name of reciprocal averaging. The iterative procedure uses the row scores to adjust the column scores which are then used to adjust the row scores and so on until the change in scores is below some preset minimum criterion. The result is a set of row and column scores that have the maximum possible correlation. This must then be repeated for all other axes but with a constraint that between-axis scores must be uncorrelated. The 'quality' of the solution can be judged from the eigen values of the axes, which can be viewed as the correlation coefficient between the row and column scores. Therefore, large eigen values indicate significant correlation that allows the axis to be used for interpretative purposes. This can be seen if the rows and columns are re-sequenced using the row and column totals. If the scores are correlated the table will develop some structure. For example, using the data from Table 1.1, Figure 2.5 shows a plot of the cases on the first two axes from a correspondence analysis. The same 'horseshoe' effect from Figure 1.1 is apparent. The row (case) and column (variable) scores, from the first axis, can be used to re-sequence the rows and columns in the table, which then reveals the structure (Table 2.4). The eigen value for the first axis is 0.54, suggesting a moderate correlation. The eigen value for the second axis is only 0.11, suggesting the presence of only very minor correlation.

The second, and preferred, algorithm for correspondence analysis uses an eigen analysis of the data matrix plus other derived matrices. Full details are given in Jongman *et al.* (1995).

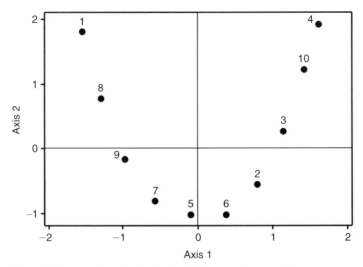

Figure 2.5 Scatter plot of axis 1 and axis 2 scores for cases from a correspondence analysis of the data in Table 2.4.

Correspondence analysis has a well-known problem, which is shared with PCA, called the arch or horseshoe effect (see Figure 2.5). This problem arises when there is a single, long gradient which results in the data points being arranged in an arched pattern along the first two axes. Detrended correspondence analysis (Hill and Gauch, 1980) overcomes this problem with a rather crude algorithm. Scores on the first axis are split into segments and the scores on the second axis are adjusted so that the mean score of the points within each segment is the same in all segments. The usual metaphor to describe the process is using a hammer to beat out the distortions in a sheet of metal.

A detailed annotated analysis of ecological applications can be found on Palmer's ordination web pages (http://ordination.okstate.edu/CA.htm).

2.7.2   Canonical correspondence analysis

When techniques such as correspondence analysis are used in ecology they are used as indirect gradient analysis methods. This means that identifiable trends in the data, such as species abundance, have to be compared to other environmental data, which were not included in the analysis, to discover the possible causes for the trends in species data. However, canonical correspondence analysis (ter Braak, 1986, 1987) is a multivariate direct gradient analysis method that has become very widely used in ecology. Direct gradient analysis methods incorporate explanatory variables, such as pH, with the species abundance data. The method is based on correspondence analysis but with a modification that

Table 2.4. *Structure in an artificial data set identified using correspondence analysis.*
The first table is the original data with row and column scores from a correspondence
analysis. The second table has rows and columns sorted using the scores from the first axis.
The third table has rows and columns sorted using the second axis scores. The zeros have
been blanked in the second and third tables to highlight the structures (if present)

Case	a	b	c	d	e	f	g	h	i	Axis 1	Axis 2
1	2	0	1	4	0	5	3	0	0	−1.552	1.814
2	2	4	3	0	5	0	1	4	3	0.792	−0.544
3	1	3	2	0	4	0	0	5	4	1.141	0.266
4	0	1	0	0	2	0	0	3	4	1.606	1.931
5	4	4	5	2	3	1	3	2	1	−0.100	−1.012
6	3	5	4	1	4	0	2	3	2	0.378	−1.014
7	5	3	4	3	2	2	4	1	0	−0.573	−0.810
8	3	1	2	5	0	4	4	0	0	−1.298	0.777
9	4	2	3	4	1	3	5	0	0	−0.970	−0.165
10	0	2	1	0	3	0	0	4	5	1.421	1.223
Axis 1	−0.429	0.303	−0.090	−0.954	0.629	−1.141	−0.716	0.897	1.112		
Axis 2	−0.278	−0.324	−0.374	0.264	−0.125	0.603	−0.051	0.180	0.538		

Case	f	d	g	a	c	b	e	h	i	Axis 1	Axis 2
1	5	4	3	2	1					−1.552	1.814
8	4	5	4	3	2	1				−1.298	0.777
9	3	4	5	4	3	2	1			−0.970	−0.165
7	2	3	4	5	4	3	2	1		−0.573	−0.810
5	1	2	3	4	5	4	3	2	1	−0.100	−1.012
6		1	2	3	4	5	4	3	2	0.378	−1.014
2			1	2	3	4	5	4	3	0.792	−0.544
3				1	2	3	4	5	4	1.141	0.266
10					1	2	3	4	5	1.421	1.223
4						1	2	3	4	1.606	1.931
Axis 1	−1.141	−0.954	−0.716	−0.429	−0.090	0.303	0.629	0.897	1.112		
Axis 2	0.603	0.264	−0.051	−0.278	−0.374	−0.324	−0.125	0.180	0.538		

Case	c	b	a	e	g	h	d	i	f	Axis 1	Axis 2
1		1		2	0	3		4		1.606	1.931
4	1		2		3		4		5	−1.552	1.814
10	1	2		3	0	4		5		1.421	1.223
8	2	1	3		4		5		4	−1.298	0.777
3	2	3	1	4		5	0	4		1.141	0.266
9	3	2	4	1	5	0	4	0	3	−0.970	−0.165
2	3	4	2	5	1	4	0	3		0.792	−0.544
7	4	3	5	2	4	1	3		2	−0.573	−0.810
6	5	4	4	3	3	2	2	1	1	−0.100	−1.012
5	4	5	3	4	2	3	1	2		0.378	−1.014
Axis 1	−0.008	0.027	−0.037	0.055	−0.059	0.074	−0.074	0.086	−0.078		
Axis 2	−0.014	−0.012	−0.010	−0.005	−0.002	0.006	0.009	0.017	0.017		

allows environmental data to be incorporated. Canonical correspondence analysis programs normally use the iterative, reciprocal averaging algorithm but with the addition of a multiple regression at each iteration. Sample scores are regressed on the environmental variables and the predicted scores are used to estimate the new site scores. The final projection has axes that are linear combinations of the environmental variables and the species data. This combination allows the changes in species abundance to be directly interpreted as responses to the environmental variables.

2.8   Other methods

2.8.1   Mantel tests

The Mantel test (Mantel, 1967) is a very useful, if somewhat obscure, test which is not widely used in biology. This is a pity because it can be used to investigate some sophisticated questions. Basically it is used to test if two distance matrices are correlated. For example, suppose that one has two distance matrices:

1. a matrix of genetic distances between populations (i.e. a measure of their genetic similarity)
2. a matrix of geographical distances (i.e. a measure of how spatially separate the populations are).

It is reasonable to ask if genetic distances are correlated with the geographical distances, i.e. do individuals become increasingly different the further apart they live? A simple correlation coefficient cannot be used because the cases are not independent (e.g. the distance between cases one and three is not independent of the distance between cases one and four because case one is involved in both).

A correlation coefficient, R_0, is calculated for the original matrices. Next the rows and columns within one of the distance matrices are permuted prior to recalculating the correlation. This is repeated hundreds, or preferably thousands, of times. If the original matrices had been correlated the disruption caused by the permutations should reduce the correlation coefficient. The significance measure is the number of times that the original correlation coefficient (R_0) was exceeded by the permutated values. For example, if there were 999 permutations (plus the original) and only one of the permutated coefficients exceeded R_0 this would be a p value of 0.001. Conversely, if the matrices were uncorrelated there is no reason to assume that the permutations would decrease the correlation coefficient; they may indeed increase it.

Legendre and Lapointe (2004) explain how a modified Mantel test can be used to compare distance matrices, derived from different variable types, to determine if they can be used together in a subsequent analysis. They use an example from an earlier paper (Lapointe and Legendre, 1994) which examines the characteristics of Scottish malt whiskies.

Some recent examples of the use of Mantel tests in biology include Stefanescu *et al.* (2005) who identified a relationship between habitat types and butterfly species, Spinks and Shaffer (2005) examined geographical and genetic variation in mitochondrial and nuclear DNA sequences while Davis (2005) found a relationship between climate and phylogenetic distance matrices in marmots.

Mantel tests are absent from most statistical packages but one is available in Hood's (2005) Poptools, a free Excel add-in. Bonnet and Van de Peer (2002) describe the test and their free zt software (http://www.psb.rug.ac.be/~erbon/mantel/). Clarke *et al.* (2002) have developed a program (DISTMAT) to extend the Mantel test to a regression-type analysis in which one distance matrix, e.g. a matrix of genetic distances, can be regressed on a predictor matrix, such as a matrix of geographical distances. Their program provides several methods that provide valid standard errors for the regression parameters and valid confidence limits for the regression relationship.

2.8.2   *Procrustes rotation*

The name derives from a story in Greek mythology. Procrustes was an innkeeper who liked to make sure that visitors fitted into their beds. Unfortunately he tended to do this by stretching people if they were too short or removing limbs if they were too tall. Consequently the name became attached to a procedure that distorts objects to make them fit.

Procrustes rotation is typically used to compare the results from different data projections. For example, two projections, possibly from multidimensional scaling analyses, may be very similar but on different projections. For example, one could be a rotation and translation of the other. In the spirit of Procrustes, the method rotates and expands or contracts axes as needed to maximise the similarity. Imagine two dice, one with a six on the top surface and the other with a one on top. If one of the dice is rotated both can have the six on top. The Procrustes rotation attempts to do something similar with matrices whose columns are the coordinates of the cases (rows). The analysis rotates one matrix, containing the coordinates from one projection, to achieve a maximum similarity with a second matrix of coordinates, measured as the sum of squared differences between the two solutions. This allows different projections to be compared after removing any rotation or translation differences.

2.9   Data dredging

It is important to note that some view EDA with suspicion and view it as 'data dredging', an uncomplimentary term which describes the hope that the EDA will generate some ideas. Instead these critics favour an information theoretic model comparison (ITMC) approach which is predicated on a priori hypotheses (of which there may be many competing forms). However, others, such as Wren *et al.* (2005), support Tukey's view that 'Finding the question is often more important than finding the answer' (from Brillinger, 2002). These opposing views are actually part of a wider debate on the relative merits of null hypothesis testing and ITMC. Stephens *et al.* (2005) debate their relative merits in an ecological context, although their arguments are much more general. They consider that it is difficult to construct the multiparameter models needed for an ITMC approach when the research is exploring a knowledge-poor problem. In these circumstances the Tukey quotation becomes relevant. As Stephens *et al.* (2005) note, 'exploration of the data using a range of graphical and statistical approaches may reveal unexpected patterns that lead to new hypotheses'. Although the ITMC approach will find the best (according to a restricted set of criteria) model from a list of candidate models this is not always the most useful at the start of the analysis cycle (see Chatfield, 1995 and Altman and Royston, 2000).

2.10   Example EDA analysis

This example uses a very well-known data set, first published by Fisher in 1936, to illustrate how exploratory methods can be used to help identify and understand patterns in data. The data set has four flower measurements (petal length and width, sepal length and width) for three species of *Iris* (*setosa, versicolor* and *virginica*). The data are available from many web sources and an online search will soon identify a suitable source.

The individual value plots in Figure 2.6 show individual values by moving points sideways if they overlap with other cases. It is apparent from this plot that there are few outliers and the three species have different means for all four variables. In general the amount of variation, within a variable, appears similar with the exception of the *I. setosa* petal measurements. The greatest separation between the species is shown with the petal measurements. However, *I. versicolor*

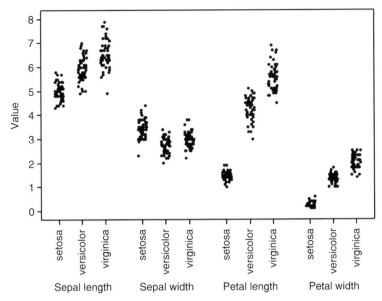

Figure 2.6 Individual value plots for the four variables from three *Iris* species.

and *I. virginica* cannot be completely separated by any of the variables. Table 2.5 provides more information as a range of summary statistics

Apart from the means, the most obvious differences between the species in Table 2.5 are the large values for the coefficient of variation and skewness for *I. setosa*. The apparent reduction in variability in petal measurements shown by *I. setosa* in Figure 2.6 is largely an artefact of the different means. Proportionally, *I. setosa* exhibits the greatest variability. Three of the nine species–variable normality tests have p values less than 0.05, suggesting a significant deviation from normality. However, the probability plots, see Figure 2.7 for an example, do not indicate that the deviations from normality will be too problematic. The Anderson–Darling test used as a goodness of fit test emphasises deviations in the tails of the distribution and, since there are few data points involved, it is unlikely that a transformation will improve the fit.

The matrix of bivariate scatter plots (Figure 2.8) clearly separates *I. setosa* from the other two species on its individual petal measurements. Although the individual sepal measurements do separate *I. setosa* from the other two species on their own, there is some evidence for a clearer separation when used in conjunction. However, *I. versicolor* and *I. virginica* show considerable overlap on all of the plots, suggesting that they cannot be separated by single, or pairs of, variables. Note that *I. setosa* has very little variation in petal length or width relative to the other two species, which means that their relationships with the

Table 2.5. *Summary statistics for each variable broken down by species. CV is the coefficient of variation. Skewness measures the presence of any skew in the data with values close to zero indicating symmetry while positive values suggest a positive or right skew. The Anderson–Darling test was used to test if the data conform to a normal distribution: if the p value is less than 0.05 this indicates a significant deviation from normality*

Species		Sepal length	Sepal width	Petal length	Petal width
I. setosa	Means	5.01	3.43	1.46	0.25
I. versicolor		5.94	2.77	4.26	1.33
I. virginica		6.59	2.97	5.55	2.03
I. setosa	Standard error	0.05	0.05	0.02	0.01
I. versicolor		0.07	0.04	0.07	0.03
I. virginica		0.09	0.05	0.08	0.04
I. setosa	CV	7.04	11.06	11.88	42.84
I. versicolor		8.70	11.33	11.03	14.91
I. virginica		9.65	10.84	9.94	13.56
I. setosa	Minimum	4.30	2.30	1.00	0.10
I. versicolor		4.90	2.00	3.00	1.00
I. virginica		4.90	2.20	4.50	1.40
I. setosa	Maximum	5.80	4.40	1.90	0.60
I. versicolor		7.00	3.40	5.10	1.80
I. virginica		7.90	3.80	6.90	2.50
I. setosa	Skewness	0.12	0.04	0.11	1.25
I. versicolor		0.11	−0.36	−0.61	−0.03
I. virginica		0.12	0.37	0.55	−0.13
I. setosa	Normality (p)	0.33	0.21	0.01	0.01
I. versicolor		0.43	0.14	0.14	0.01
I. virginica		0.15	0.10	0.11	0.06

sepal characteristics is less clear. In both *I. versicolor* and *I. virginica* the four floral characters are significantly correlated with each other but in *I. setosa* neither of the petal characters is correlated with a sepal character, although lengths and widths are correlated within sepals and petals.

Because the four floral measurements have some significant correlations it may be possible to reduce the dimensionality of these data using a PCA or MDS method. A PCA of the four variables supports this assumption with almost 96% of the variation being retained in the first two components.

```
Eigenanalysis of the Iris floral dimensions correlation matrix
Eigenvalue  2.9185  0.9140  0.1468  0.0207
Proportion  0.730   0.229   0.037   0.005
Cumulative  0.730   0.958   0.995   1.000
```

Variable	PC1	PC2	PC3	PC4
Sepal length	0.521	−0.377	−0.720	0.261
Sepal width	−0.269	−0.923	0.244	−0.124
Petal length	0.580	−0.024	0.142	−0.801
Petal width	0.565	−0.067	0.634	0.524

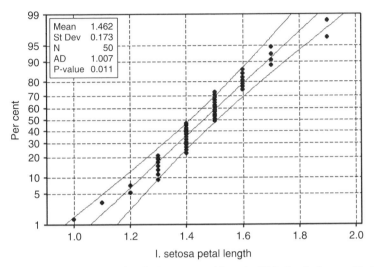

Figure 2.7 Probability plot for *I. setosa* petal length. AD is the Anderson−Darling statistic.

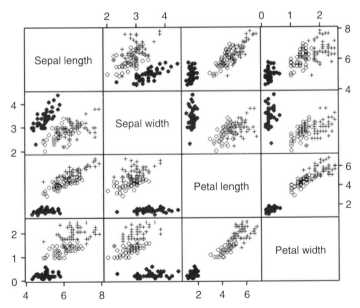

Figure 2.8 Matrix of bivariate scatter plots. *I. setosa*, filled circle; *I. versicolor*, open circle; *I. virginica*, cross.

Note that if Kaiser's rule, of only retaining components with an eigen value greater than one, was used only one component that retained 75% of the variation would be extracted. However, the second component has an eigen value (0.91) close to one and it retains almost a quarter (22.9%) of the variation. It makes sense, therefore, to extract two components.

The first component is associated with all but one of the variables. Sepal width has a relatively small loading on PC1 but is the only one with large loading on the second. Consequently, these data appear to have two effective dimensions. The first is associated with three of the floral measurements and probably reflects size differences between the flowers, while the second, which is mainly sepal width, reflects a change in the shape of the flowers.

If case scores on these new components are examined (Figure 2.9) it is very apparent that the first axis shows the biggest separation between the species reflecting the different sizes of the flowers. However, as with the individual variables, only *I. setosa* is clearly separated from the others. The second component shows that *I. versicolor* is slightly different from the other two species. The remaining two component scores are also shown in Figure 2.9. However, they would not normally be considered further because they explain so little of the original variation. These scores also show very little variation and no separation between the species.

Figure 2.10 is a scatter plot of the first two component scores. Clearly, this plot separates out the *I. setosa* individuals. However, it also highlights another important difference. The relationship between the component scores is insignificant in *I. setosa*, while the relationships in *I. versicolor* and *I. virginica* are both highly significant and negative.

Although it is not needed for this exploratory analysis, the data were also subjected to an NMDS analysis using a Euclidean distance measure. The results are shown in Figure 2.11. There is an obvious similarity between this plot and that in Figure 2.10. The only differences are translational (a reflection and an inversion). This could be verified using a Procrustes analysis. While the NMDS analysis clearly highlights the overlap between *I. versicolor* and *I. virginica*, and their separation from *I. setosa*, it is less informative because it does not provide any information about how the four variables contributed to the reduction in dimensions.

The final part of this EDA uses the GAP software (Wu and Chen, 2006) to highlight the similarities and differences between the three species using a technique that shares a lot in common with Bertin's re-orderable matrix (Section 2.4.1). Euclidean distances (Section 3.2.1) are calculated for each pair of cases. Small Euclidean distances indicate cases that have similar values for all four of the floral characters. If the Euclidean distance is large the pair of cases

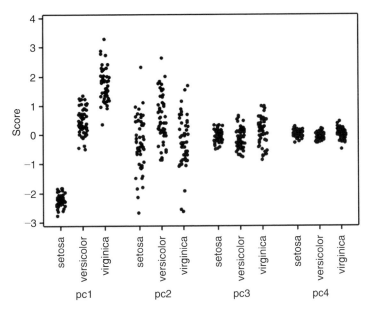

Figure 2.9 Individual value plots for the principal component scores from three *Iris* species.

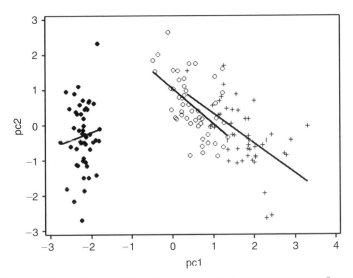

Figure 2.10 Scatter plot of the first two principal component scores from three *Iris* species. Trend lines are also shown. Symbols as in Figure 2.8.

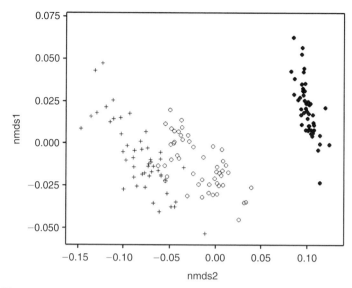

Figure 2.11 Scatter plot of the first two scores from an NMDS analysis of the floral characteristics from three *Iris* species. Symbols as in Figure 2.8.

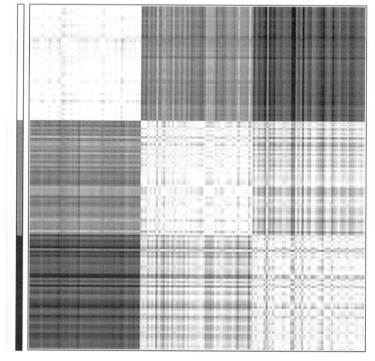

Figure 2.12 GAP plot (Wu and Chen, 2006) showing the Euclidean distance between each pair of cases. Cases are in their original order. The grey scale goes from white (identical) to black (maximum dissimilarity). The vertical bar on the left side of the plot identifies the species: *I. setosa* (white), *I. versicolor* (grey) and *I. virginica* (black).

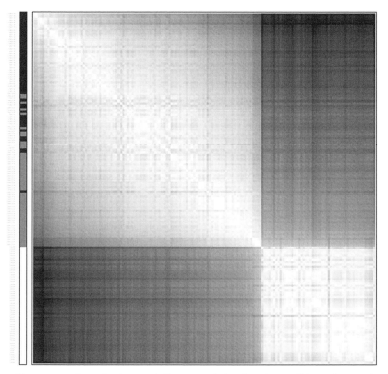

Figure 2.13 GAP plot (Wu and Chen, 2006) showing the Euclidean distance between each pair of cases. Cases are sorted using an ellipse sort. The grey scale is the same as Figure 2.12.

is dissimilar with respect to one or more of the characters. The first plot (Figure 2.12) represents the data table with cases in their original order, which includes a separation into species. The greyscale goes from white (identical) to black (maximum dissimilarity). The second plot (Figure 2.13) shows the same data but with the rows and columns reordered to highlight any structure in the data. As with all of the previous analyses the separation of *I. setosa* from the other species is confirmed, as is the overlap between the other two species.

3

Cluster analysis

3.1 Background

Cluster analysis is an approach that finds structure in data by identifying natural groupings (clusters) in the data. Unfortunately 'natural groupings' is not as well defined as we might hope. Indeed, it is usual to have more than one natural grouping for any collection of data. As we will see, there is no definitive cluster analysis technique, instead the term relates to a rather loose collection of algorithms that group similar objects into categories (clusters). Although some clustering algorithms have been present in 'standard' statistical software packages for many years, they are rarely used for formal significance testing. Instead they should be viewed as EDA tools because they are generally used to generate, rather than test, hypotheses about data structures.

A cluster is simply a collection of cases that are more 'similar' to each other than they are to cases in other clusters. This intentionally vague definition is common; for example, Sneath and Sokal (1973) noted that vagueness was inevitable given the multiplicity of different definitions while Kaufman and Rousseeuw (1990) referred to cluster analysis as the 'art of finding groups'.

If an analysis produces obvious clusters it may be possible to name them and summarise the cluster characteristics. Consequently, the biggest gains are likely in knowledge-poor environments, particularly when there are large amounts of unlabelled data. Indeed clustering techniques can be viewed as a way of generating taxonomies for the classification of objects. However, as with the well-established biological taxonomies, there will still be room for debate and disagreement about the validity of a particular taxonomy. This is reinforced by the lack of any test of accuracy. Instead, as is appropriate for an EDA method (Chapter 2), the results should be judged by their usefulness.

Obviously usefulness is in the 'eye of the beholder', a fact that should not be forgotten when promoting a particular classification over other possibilities.

Take a shuffled deck of cards as an example (shuffled at least seven times to ensure a random order). Present this to a colleague and ask them turn over the cards one by one and place them into groups (clusters). The obvious outcome is that they will be placed into the four suits (hearts, clubs, diamonds and spades), but is that the only natural grouping? Others are apparent:

- Face and number cards (two groups)
- Red and black cards (two groups)
- Card value (thirteen groups)
- Odd, even and face cards (three groups)

Arguments can be made in favour of all five of these, and other, groupings. None of them is wrong, they are just different. The solution found by an automated procedure will depend upon the criteria used in the clustering. This is important − the choice of criteria will direct the clustering along a particular path and prevent other solutions from being found. Indeed, before beginning any unsupervised clustering of unlabelled cases it is worth remembering that the algorithms will place cases into clusters, even when real clusters do not exist. This is because, in general, they do not 'give up' if there is no obvious structure. The rules continue to be applied until all cases are in clusters. Secondly, combined with the absence of a single valid solution, there is no default, best method. It is, therefore, unwise to attach too much value to the results from a single clustering exercise.

The types of clusters formed in these five playing card examples are disjoint in that a single partitioning splits the cards into two or more final clusters. There is another approach which allows for clusters to be further subdivided. An obvious example would be to initially split the cards into red and black clusters. Each of these could then be split into their suits (four clusters) and then into face and non-face cards (eight clusters). This is known as hierarchical clustering and the method creates a taxonomy of cluster relatedness.

The partitioning and hierarchical methods are two general classes of clustering methods. In fact there is a wide range of algorithms. In addition to the partitioning and hierarchical methods there are also model-, density- and grid-based methods. Grabmeier and Rudolph (2002) described one of many possible taxonomies of clustering algorithms (Figure 3.1).

In Figure 3.1 the first split separates partitioning from hierarchical approaches. The first class of methods, which use iterative approaches to partition the cases, are sub-divided on the methods by which the number of partitions is specified. In the user-defined method the number of clusters

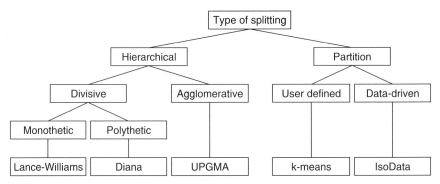

Figure 3.1 Taxonomy of clustering algorithms (simplified version of Figure 6 in Grabmeier and Rudolph, 2002). Each group has a final box listing one representative algorithm.

is specified by the analyst while other methods derive this from the data themselves. There are two major classes of hierarchical methods. Divisive methods begin with all of the cases in one cluster which is broken down into sub-clusters until all cases are separated (e.g. DIANA; Kaufman and Rousseeuw, 2005). However, the divisive approach is rarely used because of computational difficulties, although decision trees (Chapter 6) use a divisive approach to complete a supervised classification. The agglomerative approach works in the opposite direction as single-member clusters are increasingly fused (joined) until all cases are in one cluster. Chipman and Tibshirani (2005) have proposed a hybrid scheme that combines hierarchical and divisive solutions. The split of divisive methods into mono- and polythetic relates to the number of variables employed. Monothetic methods use only one variable to allocate cases to clusters while polythetic approaches use two or more.

3.2   Distance and similarity measures

3.2.1   *Distance measures*

In the playing card example clusters were formed by placing similar cards into the same cluster. All clustering algorithms begin by measuring the similarity between the cases to be clustered. Cases that are similar will be placed into the same cluster. It is also possible to view similarity by its inverse, the distance between cases, with distance declining as similarity increases. This leads to a general conclusion that objects in the same cluster will be closer to each other (more similar) than they are to objects in other clusters. It also means that there must some means of measuring distance.

There are a surprisingly large number of methods (metrics) by which distance can be measured. Some are restricted to particular data types but all share the property that distance declines with increasing similarity. However, they do not share a common distance between the same two cases, i.e. distance changes with the similarity measure – leading to the potential alternative arrangements for a deck of playing cards.

Selecting the appropriate distance metric is important because different metrics will result in different cluster memberships and a consequential change to the biological interpretation. The most obvious distances are Euclidean (straight lines that can be measured with a 'ruler') while others, often based on similarity, are non-Euclidean. For example, 'as the crow flies' (a Euclidean distance) the city of York is closer to Manchester than it is to Canterbury. However, if distance (similarity) is measured in terms of city characteristics, York is closer to Canterbury.

Three general classes of distance measures are defined below and then measures that are appropriate for different datatypes are described.

Euclidean metrics

These metrics measure true straight-line distances in Euclidean space. In a univariate example the Euclidean distance between two values is the arithmetic difference, i.e. $value_1 - value_2$. In a bivariate case the minimum distance between two points is the hypotenuse of a triangle formed from the points (Figure 3.2, Pythagoras theorem). For three variables the hypotenuse extends through three-dimensional space. Although difficult to visualise, an extension of Pythagoras theorem gives the distance between two points in n-dimensional space: distance $(a,b) = (\sum(a_i - b_i)^2)^{1/2}$.

Non-Euclidean metrics

These are distances that are not straight lines, but which obey four rules. The first three are simple, the fourth is more complex. Let d_{ij} be the distance between two cases, i and j.

d_{ij} must be 0 or positive (objects are identical, $d_{ij} = 0$, or they are different, $d_{ij} > 0$).

$d_{ij} = d_{ji}$ (the distance from A to B is the same as that from B to A).

$d_{jj} = 0$ (an object is identical to itself!).

$d_{ik} \leq d_{ij} + d_{jk}$ (when considering three objects the distance between any two of them cannot exceed the sum of the distances between the other two pairs. In other words the distances can be constructed

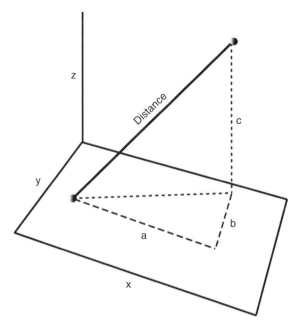

Figure 3.2 Calculating Euclidean distance in three-dimensional space. The distance between the two points is the square root of $(a^2 + b^2 + c^2)$.

as a triangle. For example, if $d_{ik} = 10$ and $d_{ij} = 3$ and $d_{jk} = 4$ it is impossible to construct a triangle, hence the distance measure would not be a non-Euclidean metric).

The Manhattan or City Block metric (Section 3.2.2) is an example of this type.

Semi-metrics

These distance measures obey the first three rules but may not obey the 'triangle' rule. The cosine measure (Section 3.2.2) is an example of this type.

3.2.2   *Importance of data types*

It is important to take account of the type of data since each has its own set of distance measures. In general there are three broad classes: interval, count and binary. It is not easy, or generally advisable, to mix data types in a cluster analysis. However, Gower's (1971) general coefficient of similarity can incorporate mixed variable types to estimate the general distance (s_{ij}) between two cases:

$$s_{ij} = \left(\Sigma w_{ijk} s_{ijk}\right) / w_{ijk}$$

where w_{ijk} is a user-defined weight for each variable and s_{ijk} is the distance between the two cases on the kth variable. Each variable has a similarity between 0 and 1 and these are summed to give the overall measure.

Distances for interval variables

Several distance measures for interval variables are available in most statistical packages. The following are the most common.

Euclidean: this is the normal Pythagoras theorem extended to the appropriate number of dimensions.

Squared Euclidean distance: the sum of the squared differences between scores for two cases on all variables, i.e. the squared length of the hypotenuse. This measure magnifies distances between cases that are further apart.

Chebychev: the absolute maximum difference, on one variable, between two cases: distance $(a,b) = $ maximum $|a_i - b_i|$. This measure examines distances across all of the variables but only uses the maximum distance. This one dimensional difference need not be constant across cases. For example, age could be used for one pair but height for another.

City Block or Manhattan distance: a distance that follows a route along the non-hypotenuse sides of a triangle. The name refers to the grid-like layout of most American cities which makes it impossible to go directly between two points. This metric is less affected by outliers than the Euclidean and squared Euclidean metrics:

$$\text{Distance}(a,b) = \Sigma|a_i - b_i|$$

Mahalanobis distance: a generalised version of a Euclidean distance which weights variables using the sample variance–covariance matrix. Because the covariance matrix is used this also means that correlations between variables are taken into account:

$$\text{Distance } (a,b) = [(a_i - b_i)^t S^{-1}(a_i - b_i)]^{1/2}$$

where S^{-1} is the inverse covariance matrix.

Cosine: the cosine of vectors of variables. This is a non-Euclidean, pattern similarity metric. The cosine of the angle between two vectors is identical to their correlation coefficient. However, unlike a normal correlation calculation the pairs of values are drawn from different variables for two cases rather than two variables from different cases. It also important to standardise the values across the two rows representing the cases. This is a local, not global, standardisation across, rather than within, variables. The standardisation is needed because a single variable, with much larger values, could produce outliers that would lead to a spurious value for the coefficient. The correlation can also be viewed as the Euclidean distance between the cases after normalising them to have a mean of zero and a standard deviation of one. Because correlation coefficients measure association and not agreement they fail to distinguish between a pair of cases which share the same values across the variables and another pair in which one set of values is a multiple of the other. For example, consider three cases A, B and C which have the values [1,2,3,4], [1,2,3,4] and [2,4,6,8] for four variables. All three are perfectly correlated with each other, but case C is widely separated from the other two in Euclidean space. The Euclidean distances are 0.0 for A and B and 5.48 for A or B against C. The consequences of these characteristics is that cosine-type measures tend to cluster cases which have a similar 'shape' rather than 'size'. The Pearson correlation coefficient is often used when clustering gene expression data. However, it is susceptible to the effects of outliers which can have a disproportionate effect on its value. Therefore, a more robust, jack-knifed version is recommended (Heyer *et al.*, 1999) which tends to minimise the effect of outliers.

Non-parametric measures: one problem with using parametric correlation coefficients is that they are sensitive to outliers. One way of retaining a similar measure, but reducing the outlier effect, is to use a non-parametric correlation. Bickel (2003) explains how these rank correlation measures can be used for robust clustering of microarray data.

Data transformations

One problem with distances is that they can be greatly influenced by variables that have the largest values. Consider the pair of points (200, 0.2 and 800, 1.0). The Euclidean distance between them is the square root of $(600^2 + 0.8^2)$, which is the square root of $(360\,000 + 0.64) = 600.0007$. Obviously this distance is almost entirely dominated by the first variable. Similarly, the Chebychev distance would almost certainly use only the first variable, making the second redundant. One way around this problem is to standardise the variables. For example, if both are forced to have a scale within the range 0–1 the two distances become 0.6 and 0.8, which are much more equitable. The value of d is then 1.0, and both variables have contributed significantly to this distance. Gordon (1999) argues that standardisation is part of a broader problem of variable weighting, with the extreme being the exclusion of a variable from the analysis.

Count data

Chi-square measure: this measure is based on the chi-square test of equality for two sets of frequencies. The chi-square distance is non-Euclidean because each squared distance is weighted by the inverse of the frequency corresponding to each term. This weighting compensates for the discrepancies in variance between high and low frequencies. Without this standardisation, the differences between larger proportions would tend to dominate the distance calculation. In other words differences between frequencies should be proportional rather than absolute.

Phi-square measure: this is the chi-square measure normalised by the square root of the combined frequency.

Binary data

There is a surprisingly large number of metrics available for binary data, for example SPSS v12.0 lists 27. It is even more confusing because many have more than one name. All of these measures use two or more of the values obtained from a simple two by two matrix of agreement.

		Case	i
		$+$	$-$
Case j	$+$	a	b
	$-$	c	d

Cell a is the number of cases which both share the attribute, while in d neither have the attribute. Cells b and c are the number of cases in which only one of the pair has the attribute. Note that $a + b + c + d = n$, the sample size.

Many of these measures differ with respect to the inclusion of double negatives (d). Is it valid to say that the shared absence of a character is indicative of similarity? The answer is that it depends on the context: sometimes it is and sometimes it is not. In particular it depends on the attribute represented by a binary variable. In some cases, e.g. presence or absence of a character, the zero has an obvious meaning, but in others, such as gender where $0 =$ male and $1 =$ female, the meaning of the zero is less obvious. Grabmeier and Rudolph (2002) differentiated between symmetric and indicative (asymmetric) binary variables. Gender, coded as 0/1, would be symmetric because the coding could be reversed without any effect on distance measures, i.e. it does not matter if a male is coded as a zero or one. Indicating variables identify if two cases share a common property, e.g. both carry a particular mutation. Reversing the coding would confound the measure of distance for an indicating variable. Any binary measure, such as those listed in Table 3.1, which includes d in its calculation assumes that joint absences are important in determining similarity. If a or d are used the index measures similarity whereas an index that uses only b and c is a measure of dissimilarity.

3.2.3   *Other distance measures*

Measuring similarity between sections of text, such as amino acid sequences, is difficult and special purpose measures are needed to cope with the consequences of gaps within one or both sequences. One of the most common measures uses the BLAST algorithm (Basic Local Alignment Search Tool, http://www.ncbi.nlm.nih.gov/blast/blast_overview.shtml). BLAST is able to cope with gaps because it uses a heuristic algorithm to look for local rather than

Table 3.1. *Nine common binary similarity and distance measures. Note that*
n = a + b + c + d

Name	Equation	Comments
Euclidean distance	SQRT($b + c$)	Square root of the sum of discordant cases, the minimum value is zero, and it has no upper limit.
Squared Euclidean distance	$b + c$	Sum of discordant cases, minimum value is zero, and it has no upper limit. This will give the same result as the Manhattan distance (also known as Hamming distance).
Pattern difference	$bc/(n^2)$	A dissimilarity measure with a range from zero to one.
Variance	$(b + c)/4n$	A dissimilarity measure that uses the discordant variables. The range is zero to one.
Simple matching	$(a + d)/n$	A similarity measure that measures the ratio of matches to the total number of values. Equal weight is given to matches and non-matches.
Dice	$2a/(2a + b + c)$	A similarity measure in which joint absences (d) are excluded from consideration, and matches (a) are weighted double. Also known as the Czekanowski or Sorensen measure.
Jaccard	$a/(a + b + c)$	A similarity measure in which joint absences are excluded from consideration. Unlike the dice coefficient, equal weight is given to matches and mismatches.
Lance and Williams	$(b + c)/(2a + b + c)$	Range of zero to one. (Also known as the Bray–Curtis non-metric coefficient.)
Simpson's	$a/\text{minimum}(b,c)$	The ratio of the number of matches and the minimum number of presences in the two cases. Two cases are identical if one is a subset of the other.

global alignments. This enables it to detect relationships among sequences that share only isolated regions of similarity. Sasson *et al.* (2002) examined the performance of various clustering algorithms to compare protein sequences using the BLAST algorithm. They found that clusters which remained consistent across different clustering algorithms tended to comply with their InterPro annotation, suggesting the existence of protein families that differ in their evolutionary conservation.

3.3   Partitioning methods

The first split in Grabmeier and Rudolph's (2002) taxonomy separated partitioning methods from hierarchical methods. Lingras and Huang (2005) suggest that partitioning methods belong to a class of cluster-based methods, unlike the object-based methods typified by hierarchical methods. The two classes relate to the method by which cluster characteristics are determined. In the object-based methods the assignment of cases to clusters defines the clusters' characteristics while the cluster-based methods assign weight vectors to the clusters.

Partitioning methods address the problem of dividing n cases, described by p variables, into a small number (k) of discrete classes.

3.3.1   k-means

The k-means algorithm, which is one of the most frequently used, is a remarkably simple and efficient algorithm. There are two steps that are repeated (iterated) until a solution is found.

1. Begin with an initial partition into k clusters. The initial clusters could be random or based on some 'seed' values.
2. Re-partition the cases by assigning each case to the nearest cluster centre.
3. Recalculate the cluster centres as centroids.
4. Repeat steps two and three until an endpoint is reached. The endpoint will be an optimum of the criterion function.

Many of these iterative, partitioning approaches, including k-means, use a within-groups sum of squares criterion to minimise the within-cluster variation. The problem is that a true optimum partition of cases can only be found if all possible partitions (a very large number) have been examined. Because this is impossible heuristic algorithms are used that should find a good, but not necessarily the best, partition. Most partitioning methods depend on a user-supplied value for k. The square-error criterion is then applied so that the total squared error, across all k clusters, is minimised for that value of k. It is quite likely that a smaller total square-error can be achieved for a different value of k.

This algorithm tends to produce acceptable results, particularly when the clusters are compact, well-separated, hyperspheres (spheres in three-dimensional space). However, this does mean that it is not very good at finding sub-classes that are nested within larger classes. Estivill-Castro and Yang (2004) provide a detailed critique of the k-means algorithm and suggest alternatives based on medians rather than means. Briefly, they list the main problems of the k-means method as: a tendency to converge on poor local optimum; sensitivity to scaling and other transformations; sensitivity to noise and outliers; bias (converges to the wrong parameter values). However, the main problem is determining a suitable value for k.

Because the algorithm is not guaranteed to find the best partitioning it is quite possible that two runs using the same data will produce different cluster solutions. If several repeat analyses are tried the 'best' will be the one with the smallest sum of the within-cluster variances. Similarly, the analysis could be re-run with a large number of bootstrapped samples. The cluster integrity can be tested by examining how many times cases share the same cluster. An alternative approach, which appears to improve the performance of k-means clustering, is to use the results from a hierarchical cluster analysis to place the cases into initial clusters.

One big advantage of k-means clustering over other methods is that it can be used to assign new cases to the existing clusters. This is possible because the space occupied by the clustering variables is partitioned into Thiessen polygons (also known as Dirichlet tessellation). This type of partitioning splits the variable space into polygons whose boundaries are drawn perpendicular to the mid-point between two cluster centres. Therefore, any point falling within a Thiessen polygon should be assigned to that cluster. This is illustrated in Figure 3.3.

Schmelzer (2000) used k-means clustering to identify biogeographic regions whose characteristics were then correlated with monk seal *Monachus schauinlandi* abundance. In order to overcome the k-mean's shortcomings Schmelzer truncated his standardised values to a z value of 2.25. This helped to reduce the impact of outliers on the classification. Aronow *et al.* (2001) used k-means to divide dynamically regulated genes into nine kinetic pattern groups.

3.3.2   k-medians and PAM

Other partitioning methods use different averages such as medians. The advantage of using medians to define cluster centres is that they are little affected by outliers. However, it is a computationally intensive method and the faster PAM (partition around medoids) approximation method tends to suffer when the data are noisy. The PAM algorithm first computes k representative objects, called medoids and each cluster centre is constrained to be one of the observed data points. These are defined as the cases within the clusters, whose average dissimilarity to all other cases in the cluster is minimal. PAM is said to be more robust than k-means, because it minimises a sum of dissimilarities instead

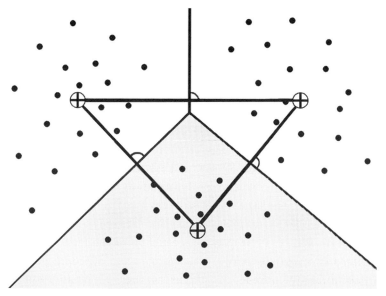

Figure 3.3 Thiessen polygons and k-means partitioning. Cases are filled circles and cluster centres are circles with a cross. The lower Thiessen is shaded grey. Any data point falling in this grey area would be assigned to that cluster.

of squared Euclidean distances. Because the algorithm can be used with any distance matrix it can be applied to more general data types than the k-means algorithm.

3.3.3   Mixture models

Mixture models, usually based on the EM (expectation maximisation) algorithm, use an alternative model-based approach, which contrasts with the heuristic data-driven approach of k-means and hierarchical clustering algorithms. Model-based approaches assume that the data are drawn from a mixture of underlying probability distributions. This enables the use of maximum likelihood methods to maximise the probability that a case belongs to a particular cluster, where the cluster is defined by a specified mixture of probability distributions. Each cluster's mixture is a multivariate probability distribution, typically multivariate normal. A multivariate normal distribution is characterised by a vector of means and a covariance matrix which, in combination, describe the geometric features of the distribution (location and shape in multivariate space). The main difficulty that has to be solved is estimating the values of the coefficients of the covariance matrix. Despite the computational difficulties the mixture-based models have the advantage that Bayesian methods can be used to determine which value of k (within a specified range) represents the best number of clusters for the data. Autoclass (Cheeseman and Stutz, 1996; available from http://ic.arc.nasa.gov/ic/projects/bayes-group/autoclass/) is a public domain mixture modelling classifier that can be used to select the most probable classification *given* the data. As with many applications of Bayes methods there is an assumption, which is almost always untrue, of independence of the predictors within a class. If the predictors are continuous a normal distribution is used, otherwise a general discrete distribution is used if the predictors are discrete. The result is a fuzzy classification, with cases assigned a probability of class membership. Riordan (1998) used Autoclass to assign correctly tiger footprints to individuals when no information was provided about the individuals. Although the aim was to develop a technique that could be used in the field with unknown animals, this preliminary study used known animals so that the performance of the classifiers could be validated. Autoclass was able to discriminate successfully between the prints from different animals and it correctly identified the number of animals, i.e. the appropriate value for k was found.

3.3.4   *Others*

The self-organising map (SOM) algorithm devised by Kohonen (1990) is a different type of partitioning algorithm that is usually found in the neural network section of books. The major difference, apart from the computational details, is that the clusters are arranged in space, typically two-dimensional, so that neighbouring clusters are similar to each other. As with tradition elsewhere, further details are provided in Chapter 6 that deals with artificial neural networks. SOMs have been quite widely used in gene expression studies. For example, Golub *et al.* (1999) successfully used a SOM to group 38 leukaemia samples on the basis of 6817 gene expression levels.

3.4   Agglomerative hierarchical methods

Partitioning methods produce a flat allocation of cases to clusters which, with the exception of a SOM, provides no additional information on the relatedness of cases. Although methods such as k-means have advantages relating to computational efficiency and an ability to classify new cases, they suffer from two main problems. Firstly, there is the need to pre-specify a value for k and, secondly, because an iterative algorithm that starts with random locations is used, the solution is not unique. The alternative hierarchical clustering paradigm does not suffer from the need to pre-specify k and it provides a visual representation (dendrogram) that highlights the relationships between cases at coarse and fine scales. However, as explained below, the solution is very dependent on the choice of algorithm and distance measure and there is no easy way to identify the number of 'major' groups that would equate to the value of k. Nonetheless, it is a very efficient tool for organising data into groups. For example, Kaplan *et al.* (2005) used hierarchical clustering to produce a taxonomy for over one million protein sequences. As should be expected with such a large dataset some of the clusters are biologically irrelevant. However, using a cluster stability index, and relevance to existing database functional annotations, 78% of the clusters could be assigned names with confidence. They also use a reordered matrix to provide evidence for sub-groups within a cluster.

3.4.1   *Joining clusters: clustering algorithms*

Hierarchical cluster analysis involves two important decisions. The first decision, which was covered in the previous section, is the selection of an appropriate distance measure. Once this has been selected a distance matrix, containing all pairwise distances between cases, can be calculated as the starting point for the second phase which begins with each case in a cluster by itself. The second stage to the clustering process is choosing the clustering or linkage algorithm, i.e. the rules which govern how distances are measured between clusters and then used to fuse clusters. As with the distance measures, there are many methods available. The criteria used to fuse clusters differ between the algorithms and hence different classifications may be obtained for the same data, even using the same distance measure. This is important because it highlights the fact that, although a cluster analysis may provide an objective method for the clustering of cases, there may be subjectivity in the choice of the analysis details. Fortunately, it appears that most combinations of distance measure and algorithm are compatible. Lance and Williams (1967) investigated this question and found that only the centroid and Ward's algorithm had a distance measure constraint. Only Euclidean distance metrics are recommended for both.

Although there are a large number of linkage algorithms most can be illustrated using five algorithms. (Figure 3.4)

Average linkage clustering

The distance between clusters is calculated using average values. However, there are many ways of calculating an average. The most common (and recommended if there is no reason for using other methods) is UPGMA (unweighted pair-groups method average). The average distance is calculated from the distance between each point in a cluster and all other points in

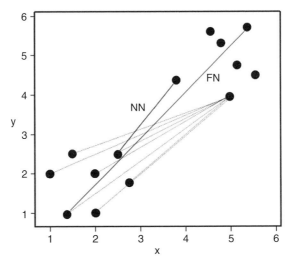

Figure 3.4 Diagrammatic summary of three clustering algorithms. NN, nearest neighbour; FN, furthest neighbour. The remaining lines illustrate how distance is measured for the UPGMA algorithm, although only the distances for one case are shown.

another cluster. The two clusters with the lowest average distance are joined together to form the new cluster.

There are other methods based on centroid and median averages. Centroid, or UPGMC (unweighted pair-groups method centroid), clustering uses the cluster centroid as the average. The centroid is defined as the centre of a cloud of points and is calculated as the weighted average point in the multidimensional space. A problem with the centroid method is that some switching and reversal may take place, for example as the agglomeration proceeds some cases may need to be switched from their original clusters. This makes interpretation of the dendrogram quite difficult.

There are weighted variations to these algorithms that use cluster size (number of cases) as a weight and they are recommended when cluster sizes are very heterogeneous.

Complete linkage clustering

In complete linkage clustering (also known as the maximum or furthest-neighbour method) the distance between clusters i and j is the greatest distance between a member of cluster i and a member of cluster j. This method tends to produce very tight clusters of similar cases and performs well when cases form distinct clusters. If the cases are more loosely spread the next algorithm may be better.

Single linkage clustering

In complete linkage clustering (also known as the minimum or nearest-neighbour method) the distance between clusters i and j is the minimum distance between members of the two clusters. This method produces long chains which form loose, straggly clusters. This method has been widely used in numerical taxonomy.

Within-groups clustering

This is similar to UPGMA except that clusters are fused so that the within-cluster variance is minimised. This tends to produce tighter clusters than the UPGMA method. This approach means that distances between clusters are not calculated.

Ward's method

Cluster membership is assessed by calculating the total sum of squared deviations from the mean of a cluster. The criterion for fusion is that it should produce the smallest possible increase in the error sum of squares. This approach means that distances between clusters are not calculated.

3.4.2   *The dendrogram*

The results of a hierarchical cluster analysis are best viewed in a graphical form known as a dendrogram. A dendrogram is a tree that shows, via its bifurcations, how clusters are related to each other across a series of scales.

Understanding how a dendrogram is constructed, and how it should be interpreted, is one of the most important aspects of cluster analysis. The calculations, and the resultant dendrogram, depend on the distance measure and/or clustering algorithm. The process is demonstrated by a simple example that ignores a lot of 'messy' details. The data set has five cases and two variables (v1 and v2).

case	v1	v2
1	1	1
2	2	1
3	4	5
4	7	7
5	5	7

A simple Euclidean distance matrix is calculated as the starting point. For example, the distance between cases three and four is the square root of $((4 - 7)^2 + (5 - 7)^2)$, which is 3.6. Only the lower triangle of the distance matrix is shown below because the distance between cases i and j is the same as that between cases j and i. Distances are presented with two significant figures. Using these distances the most similar pair of cases are one and two.

```
    1     2     3     4     5
1   0.0
2   1.0   0.0
3   5.0   4.5   0.0
4   8.5   7.8   3.6   0.0
5   7.2   6.7   2.2   2.0   0.0
```

These two cases are fused to form the first cluster. Distances must now be calculated between this cluster and the other cases. There is no need to recalculate other distances because they will not have changed. For the purpose of this exercise assume that distances are calculated from the means of v1 and v2, i.e. mean $v1_A = 1.5$, mean $v2_A = 1.0$. This produces a revised distance matrix in which cases one and two are replaced by A, the first cluster.

```
    A     3     4     5
A   0.0
3   4.7   0.0
4   8.1   3.6   0.0
5   6.9   2.2   2.0   0.0
```

The smallest distance in this matrix is between cases four and five (distance $= 2.0$). These cases are fused to form cluster B (means: $v1_B = 6$, $v2_B = 7$) and the distances are recalculated.

```
    A     B     3
A   0.0
B   7.5   0.0
3   4.7   2.8   0.0
```

The new smallest distance (2.8) is between cluster B and case three. Case three is fused with cluster B and cluster B now has three members. The mean values are: $v1_C = (4 + 5 + 7)/3 = 5.3$, $v2_C = (5 + 7 + 7)/3 = 6.3$. Obviously, there are now only two clusters and they must be the next to be fused at a distance of 6.4.

The entire process of fusions is summarised by the dendrogram (Figure 3.5). The vertical axis is the distance at which clusters were fused and the horizontal lines link fused clusters. The vertical lines, joining the links, illustrate the hierarchical nature of the fusions.

3.5   How many groups are there?

Apart from representing a possible taxonomy of relatedness between the cases, the dendrogram may also provide some evidence to answer two

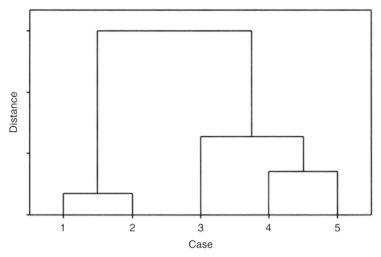

Figure 3.5 Dendrogram for simple dataset, identifying two major clusters.

fundamental questions that need to be answered after, and to a certain extent before, completing a cluster analysis. The two questions are: are the clusters real and how many clusters are there? There have been many, but no universally accepted, suggestions for approaches to these questions. Milligan and Cooper (1985) compared 30 methods for estimating the number of clusters using four hierarchical clustering methods. The best criterion that they found was a pseudo F-statistic developed by Calinski and Harabasz (1974). The Calinski–Harabasz index measures the separation between clusters and is calculated as $S_b/(k-1)/S_w/$ $(n-k)$, where S_b is the sum of squares between the clusters, S_w the sum of squares within the clusters, k the number of clusters and n the number of observations. The value of the index increases with the separation between groups. Therefore, it is possible to plot a graph of the index against the number of clusters and identify the optimum for k. However, as Pillar (1999) points out the Milligan and Cooper (1985) tests used simulated data with well-separated clusters. Pillar (1999) devised a computationally intensive alternative measure that uses a general bootstrap procedure to measure the similarity between solutions.

3.5.1   Scree plots

Although the Calinski–Harabasz and Pillar indices are useful, they are not generally available and may require significant computing. The scree plot is a simple alternative. It appears, from the dendrogram in Figure 3.5, that the data can be represented by two clusters: A (cases one and two) and B (cases three, four and five). However, as the number of cases increases it may not be so obvious and visual assessment of the dendrogram is likely to become increasingly subjective.

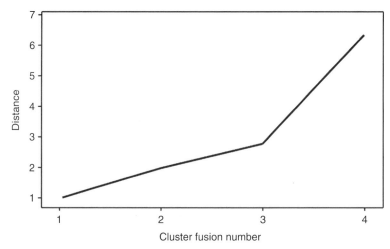

Figure 3.6 Scree plot based on the analysis in Figure 3.5.

In a hierarchical analysis, increasingly dissimilar clusters must be merged as the cluster fusion process continues. Consequently, the classification is likely to become increasingly artificial. A graph of the level of similarity at fusion versus the number of clusters may help to recognise the point at which clusters become artificial because there will be a sudden jump in the level of similarity as dissimilar groups are fused. Figure 3.6 is derived from the previous analysis. Note how there is a large jump when clusters A and B are fused. This supports the hypothesis that the data are best represented by two clusters. Tibshirani *et al.* (2001) present a more formal test of the use of the scree plot as represented by their GAP statistic, which they suggest outperforms other measures.

3.5.2   *Other methods of estimating optimum number of clusters*

Geometrical projection techniques such as PCA (Section 2.5.2) and MDS (Section 2.6) can be used as a visual check. In general these methods produce a low-dimensional (typically two or three) representation of the data such that similar cases are close together in the lower dimensional projections. However, unlike the clustering algorithms there are no explicit cluster assignments. Nonetheless cases can be plotted with cluster labels to visualise the integrity of a clustering solution. In a similar way the low-dimensional projection could be used to guide the selection of an appropriate value for k in a partitioning analysis.

In a PAM analysis each cluster can be represented by a silhouette plot which identifies cases within a cluster and those that are intermediate between two or more clusters. If all of the silhouettes are potted together the quality of the clusters can be compared. Silhouettes are constructed by calculating $s(i)$ (range

+1 to −1) values for all i cases. These are an indication of the quality of a case's assignment to a cluster. If $s(i)$ is close to +1 then case i has a much smaller dissimilarity with cases within its current cluster, compared to its dissimilarity with cases in the nearest alternative. Hence it is in the correct cluster. Alternatively, if $s(i)$ is close to −1 then case i has a larger dissimilarity with cases within its current cluster, compared to its dissimilarity with cases in the nearest alternative cluster. It must therefore be in the wrong cluster. If $s(i)$ is close to zero the case would be equally placed in two clusters.

The silhouette plot of a cluster is organised by ranking the $s(i)$ values in decreasing order. Each case is drawn as a horizontal line, with a length proportioned to $s(i)$. The average silhouette width of the silhouette plot across all clusters is the average of $s(i)$ over all cases. Therefore, a wide silhouette indicates large $s(i)$ values and hence a pronounced cluster. Because the entire silhouette plot shows the silhouettes of all clusters next to each other the quality of clusters can be compared. If the PAM is run with several values of k the resulting silhouette plots can be compared. Because larger $s(i)$ values are associated with 'better' clusters the average silhouette width can be used to select the 'best' number of clusters. The maximum average $s(i)$ value can be used as a clustering criterion. It has been suggested that a strong structure will produce a value above 0.7, while a value below 0.5 suggests that the structure is weak. If the largest mean $s(i)$, over all tested values of k, is less than 0.25 then there is little evidence for any structure.

3.6   Divisive hierarchical methods

Divisive hierarchical methods recursively partition the data in a manner that is reminiscent of the decision trees described in Chapter 6. However, the divisive hierarchical methods are unsupervised meaning that there is no 'trainer' guiding the partitioning to ensure maximum separation of pre-defined classes. Instead, it is hoped that the resulting divisions of the data will provide some information about structures within the data.

Divisive hierarchical methods do not appear to be widely used in biological applications, almost certainly because of the computational difficulties of finding the optimum partitions. TSVQ (tree structured vector quantisation) combines k-means clustering with a tree-like divisive method. k-means clustering is used to split the data into two sets, which are then recursively split using the same k-means procedure.

Two-way indicator species analysis (TWINSPAN) was developed by Hill (1979) specifically for the hierarchical classification of community data and has quite wide usage in vegetation ecology. The output is a table in which the rows (species) and columns (samples) are arranged to highlight patterns of vegetation structure. In this respect it is another example of Bertin's reorderable matrix (Section 2.5.1). It is a more complex analysis than the TSVQ algorithm and begins with a correspondence analysis. The results of this are used to split the data into two parts. The hierarchical nature of the classification is achieved by using discriminant analyses to further sub-divide each part. The most unusual part of the algorithm is the concept of a pseudo-species. This is necessary because quantitative abundance data have to be converted into presence–absence data. However, in an attempt to retain information about the relative abundances, the data are split into pseudo-species, which means that a single species may be represented by a number of pseudo-species. Hill and Šmilauer (2005) have recently made a Windows version of TWINSPAN available for download. Included with the download is a manual which provides more background on the algorithm and the interpretation of the output.

Because divisive clustering methods are better at finding large clusters than hierarchical methods, Chipman and Tibshirani (2005) used a hybrid method that also used the ability of hierarchical methods to find small clusters. Before the results from the two algorithms could be combined it was necessary to define a concept that they called a mutual cluster, which is a group of points that are sufficiently close enough to each other, and far enough from others, that they should never be separated. The small mutual clusters, identified from the hierarchical clustering, were placed into a broader context identified by the divisive clustering using the TSVQ algorithm. They demonstrated the approach using breast cancer data which has 85 tissue samples and 456 cDNA expression values.

3.7   Two-way clustering and gene shaving

Microarray data generally consist of hundreds, and possibly thousands, of gene expression levels obtained from a much smaller number of samples that come from different cell lines or timed samples that may represent different developmental phases. If it is assumed that the gene expression patterns provide important information about the cell states it is clear that some method is needed to identify the patterns. Although the clustering methods described earlier can be very useful, it is possible to use two-way clustering as a means of clarifying the patterns visually. Tibshirani *et al.* (1999) suggest that two-way clustering can discover large-scale structures but may not be as effective with fine detail.

A two-way clustering carries out simultaneous clustering, which is usually hierarchical, of the rows (gene expressions) and columns (samples) of the data matrix. In other words, the two dendrograms are generated in which the data matrix is effectively transposed. The dendrograms are used to reorder the rows and columns of the data matrix prior to using a colour scale to represent the expression level. The example in Section 3.9.1 illustrates two-way clustering using the Wu and Chen (2006) GAP software. Bryan (2004) raises a note of concern about gene clustering because she feels that the clusters are often a consequence of pre-filtering processes that tend to create structures where they were previously weak.

Tibshirani *et al.* (1999) and Hastie *et al.* (2000) describe a two-way clustering that they call gene shaving. The motivation for this approach is that the two-way clustering produces a single ordering of the samples, while more complex patterns may exist that depend on the set of genes used in the clustering. Their method begins by finding the linear combination of genes that have maximal variation among the samples. This is the first principal component of gene expression levels. This group of genes is called a 'super gene' and genes which are uncorrelated with the first principal component are removed, or shaved, from the data. The process is repeated, producing smaller and smaller clusters of size k, until only one gene remains. A gap statistic (the difference between the mean within-cluster sum of squares and the within-cluster sum of squares for a cluster of size k) is used to determine the optimum cluster size (maximum value for the gap statistic). Each row in the data matrix is then orthogonalised with respect to the average gene in the kth cluster. The process is repeated to find the second, third and mth optimal cluster, where m is pre-selected. The end result is a sequence of blocks of genes that contain similar genes with a large variance across the samples. Hastie *et al.* (2000) illustrate the use of this approach to analyse gene expression measurements from patients with diffuse large B-cell lymphoma and identified a small cluster of genes whose expression is highly predictive of survival.

3.8   Recommended reading

There are a number of general texts but amongst the most useful are Gordon (1981, 1999) and Everitt *et al.* (2001). The earlier book by Gordon is still worth reading because it is wide ranging and clearly written with a minimum of mathematical notation. The 1999 book has an additional large section on cluster validation. Everitt *et al.* (2001) is also comprehensive, with a similar 'light' mathematical touch. Their second chapter, on visualising clusters, is particularly useful as is their chapter eight which includes a section on comparing cluster solutions. Kaufman and Rousseeuw (2005) describe a number of clustering algorithms, including PAM that are implemented in the free WinIDAMS software that can be ordered from UNESCO (http://www.unesco.org/webworld/idams, visited on 4 October 2005).

Lapointe and Legendre (1994) in a wonderfully informative paper describe how a constraint, in their case spatial, can be applied to a cluster analysis. In addition to the constrained clustering they also explain how Mantel tests (Section 2.8.1) can be used to compare distance matrices derived from different sets of clustering variables. The paper also has the advantage of telling us more about the finer qualities of Scottish malt whiskies! Tibshirani *et al.* (1999) is a very useful review of clustering methods for the analysis of DNA microarray data. They also describe two-way clustering and introduce the concept of gene shaving. Bryan (2004) is a very useful review of the use of clustering methods to group genes, rather than cases, using expression data. She notes that the identified clusters are often a consequence of earlier filtering methods and that genomic-wide clusterings often fail to find discrete groups.

3.9   Example analyses

Hierarchical and partitioning clustering methods are illustrated using some small data sets. The first analyses highlight the effect of changing the distance and linkage measures on the structure of the dendrogram, and subsequent biological interpretation, from a hierarchical cluster analysis. The second set of analyses use *k*-means clustering to investigate the structure of two sets of data.

3.9.1   *Hierarchical clustering of bacterial strains*

The data are part of a data set described by Rataj and Schindler (1991). Data are presented for six species, most having data for more than one strain and sixteen binary phenotypic characters (0 = absent, 1 = present). The species are: *Escherichia coli* (ecoli), *Salmonella typhi* (styphi), *Klebsiella pneumoniae* (kpneu), *Proteus vulgaris* (pvul), *P. morganii* (pmor) and *Serratia marcescens* (smar). The data are in Appendix C. Classifications resulting from the use of two binary similarity measures and two clustering algorithms are shown (Figures 3.7 and 3.8) to illustrate the dependency of the solution on the choice of method. The main difference between the simple measures is the treatment of double zeros. In the simple matching coefficient analysis double zeros count towards the similarity while they are not used by the Jaccard coefficient.

Despite the different methods there is some consistency in these results. In particular the *Klebsiella* (kpneu) samples are consistently separated from the others and the *Proteus vulgaris* (pvul) and *P. morganii* (pmor) samples are always associated in one cluster. The most obvious differences are between the two

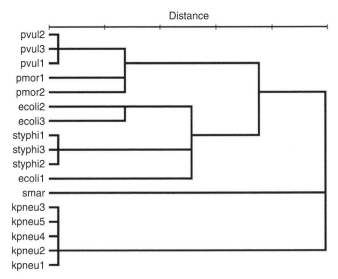

Figure 3.7 Clustering results for the bacteria data using the simple matching similarity measure and the single linkage (nearest neighbour) algorithm.

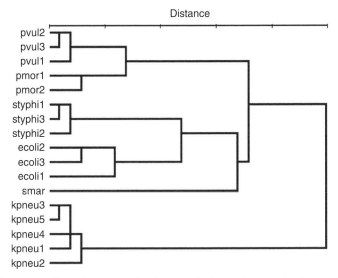

Figure 3.8 Clustering results for the bacteria data using the simple matching similarity measure and the UPGMA algorithm.

single linkage dendrograms, with the Jaccard coefficient producing a less clear-cut solution. Also, the Jaccard measure (Figure 3.9) splits the *Escherichia coli* (ecoli) and *Salmonella typhi* (styphi) samples that are clustered together in the other two analyses.

Using the GAP software (Wu and Chen, 2006) it is possible simultaneously to cluster the taxa and the variables. Using the dendrograms the data can

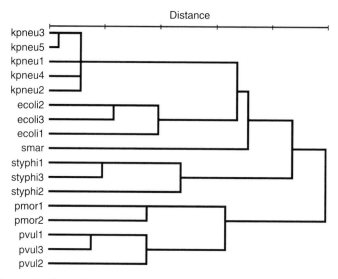

Figure 3.9 Clustering results for the bacteria data using the Jaccard similarity
measure and the single linkage (nearest neighbour) algorithm.

be ordered so that structures in both analyses are highlighted. Figures 3.10
and 3.11 show the results of the two cluster analyses using the GAP software.
Both analyses use the complete linkage algorithm but with the simple matching
and Jaccard similarity measures. The intensity of the shading is a measure
of the distance between a pair of cases with black indicating identical cases.
The box in the lower left shows the pattern of positive values for the variables,
ordered according to the clustering of the variables, i.e. which variables tended
to be jointly positive. As with the previous analyses, the *Klebsiella* (kpneu)
samples are consistently separated from the others and the *Proteus vulgaris* (pvul)
and *P. morganii* (pmor) samples are always associated in one cluster. The shading
highlights the similarity and differences between the taxonomic groups and
shows that the separation is clearer cut in Figure 3.11. One feature of the
variables is common to both plots. Four of the variables (ORN, PHE, LIP and
H2S) appear to have different profiles from the other variables. In Figure 3.10
all four are placed in a separate cluster while in Figure 3.11, which does
not use joint absences to measure similarity, they are split into two obviously
separate groups (ORN–LIP and PHE–H2S).

3.9.2   *Hierarchical clustering of the human genus*

This analysis uses data from table 5 in Wood and Collard (1999).
There are twelve gnathic variables from eight taxa related to the present
day *Homo sapiens*. Wood and Collard conclude that *Homo habilis* and *H. rudolfensis*

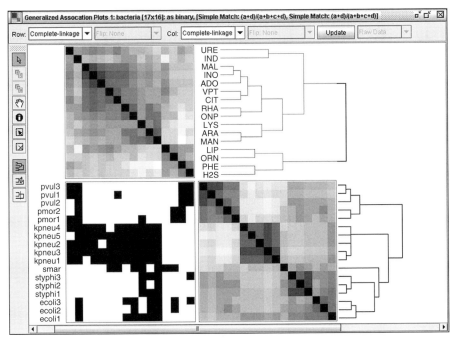

Figure 3.10 Generalised association plots for the bacterial data. A complete linkage algorithm with the simple matching coefficient was used. The intensity of shading indicates the similarity (white equals none and black equals identical).

do not belong in the genus and that the earliest taxa to satisfy the criteria are *H. ergaster* or early African *H. erectus*. The data are in Appendix D.

Two analyses are presented. Both use the UPGMA algorithm but with different distance measures. The first uses squared Euclidean distance while the second uses the cosine measure. The major difference here is that the cosine measure clusters cases which have a similar 'shape' rather than 'size', which is favoured by Euclidean distance.

Paranthropus boisei, which was previously in the *Australopithecus* genus, is an obvious outlier in the first analysis (Figure 3.12), and is well separated from *Paranthropus robustus* and *Australopithecus africanus*. However, in the second analysis (Figure 3.12), which is based on shape rather than size differences, both *Parathropus* taxa are close together along with the possibly related *Australopithecus africanus*. The three closely related *Homo* species (*sapiens, erectus* and *neanderthalensis*) are consistently close together, suggesting a similarity in both shape and size. Indeed there is debate about the appropriate taxonomic relationships, for example *H. neanderthalensis* is sometimes considered to be a sub-species of *H. sapiens*. The two taxa, *H. habilis* and *H. rudolfensis*, that Wood and Collard (1999) think should not be in the genus, are consistently well separated from *H. sapiens*,

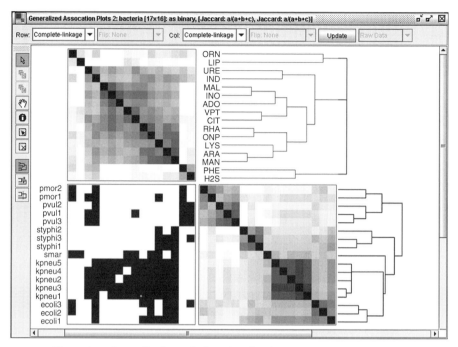

Figure 3.11 Generalised association plots for the bacterial data. A complete linkage algorithm with the Jaccard similarity coefficient was used. The intensity of shading indicates the similarity (white equals none and black equals identical).

H. erectus and *H. neanderthalensis*. These analyses demonstrate the importance of deciding on the appropriate distance metric. In particular, should similarity be measured by size or shape differences?

If the predictor data are subjected to a MDS (Figure 3.13) the pattern of taxa is broadly related to the views expressed by Wood and Collard (1999), with the three closely related *Homo* species being separated from the other taxa. The only exception is the proximity of *H. ergaster*, which is thought by some to be the same species as the adjacent *H. erectus*. The two taxa queried by Wood and Collard (1999) are close to the *Paranthropus* and *Australopithecus* taxa.

3.9.3   Partition clustering

Bacteria data

This analysis uses the data from Section 3.9.1 in which the *Klebsiella* (kpneu) samples were consistently separated from the other samples and the *Proteus vulgaris* (pvul), *P. morganii* (pmor) samples were always associated in one cluster. In this illustrative example *k* was set to six, the same as the number of taxonomic classes, but one more than the number of genera. The results are summarised in Tables 3.2 and 3.3.

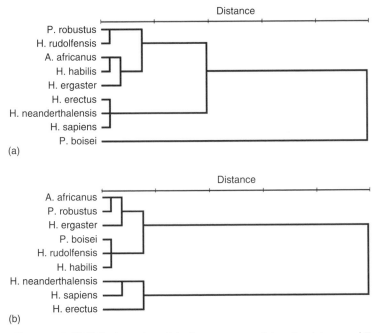

(a)

(b)

Figure 3.12 UPGMA clustering of the human genus data using (a) squared Euclidean distance measure and (b) cosine distance measure.

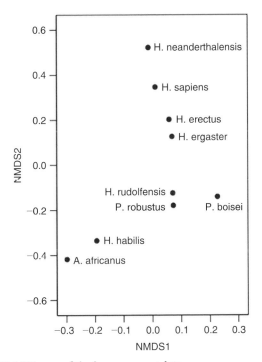

Figure 3.13 MDS map of the human genus data.

Samples have been clustered according to taxon, the only exception being the first *P. morganii* sample which is placed by itself in cluster four. However, the between-cluster distances (Table 3.3) show that clusters three and four are relatively close to each other. This is reenforced if the between-cluster distances are subjected to a MDS analysis (Figure 3.14). The results of the MDS analysis also highlights the fact that the *Klebsiella* samples are separated from the others (cluster six), while the *Escherichia coli* (ecoli), *Salmonella typhi* samples are relatively

Table 3.2. k-*means* (k = 6) *cluster results. Cluster is the cluster number assigned to each sample and distance is the distance of a case to the cluster centre*

Sample	Cluster	Distance
ecoli1	1	1.054
ecoli2	1	0.882
ecoli3	1	0.882
styphi1	5	0.471
styphi2	5	0.745
styphi3	5	0.745
kpneu1	6	0.872
kpneu2	6	0.872
kpneu3	6	0.400
kpneu4	6	0.872
kpneu5	6	0.872
pvul1	3	0.968
pvul2	3	0.661
pvul3	3	0.661
pmor1	4	0.000
pmor2	3	1.199
smar	2	0.000

Table 3.3. k-*means* (k = 6) *cluster results: distances between the cluster centres*

Cluster	1	2	3	4	5	6
1	0	2.472	2.284	2.472	1.856	2.381
2	2.472	0	2.990	2.828	2.357	2.821
3	2.284	2.990	0	1.561	2.235	3.193
4	2.472	2.828	1.561	0	2.357	3.156
5	1.856	2.357	2.235	2.357	0	2.790
6	2.381	2.821	3.193	3.156	2.790	0

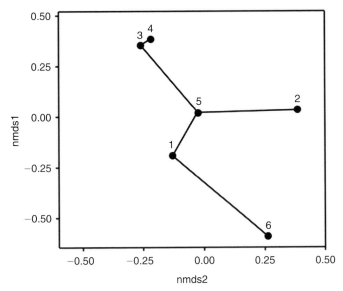

Figure 3.14 Multidimensional scaling map of the between-cluster distances from Table 3.3. Points are labelled with their cluster numbers and joined by a minimum spanning tree.

similar (clusters one and five). It is worth reinforcing the point that this analysis used only the k-means distance matrix. Raw case data were not used, unlike the analysis in Figure 3.13.

Cancer data

This analysis uses data downloaded from http://stats.math.uni-augsburg. de/Klimt/down.html (3 January 2006). The original source is Mangasarian and Wolberg (1990). There are nine continuous potential predictor variables plus one class variable (benign, malignant). The predictors are: clump thickness; uniformity of cell size; uniformity of cell shape; marginal; single epithelial cell size; bare nuclei; bland chromatin; nucleoli; and mitoses. Cases with missing values were not used in these analyses. The aim of these analyses was to determine if this unsupervised classification was capable of separating the classes using all nine of the potential predictors, but excluding the class. Three values of k were tested: two, three and four.

In all four analyses (Tables 3.4, 3.5 and 3.6) there was good separation of the classes, even though the class label was not used in the analyses. In general, the clusters containing mainly malignant class have larger means for all predictors. However, it seems from the first two analyses that the malignant class is rather heterogeneous. While the benign cases tend to be restricted to one cluster, which includes a small number of malignant cases, the malignant cases are relatively

Table 3.4. *Cluster centres and cluster class composition for* k = 4

	Cluster 1	Cluster 2	Cluster 3	Cluster 4
Clump	7	7	7	3
UnifCellSize	8	4	9	1
UnifCellsHhape	8	5	8	1
MargAdhesion	6	4	7	1
SECSize	6	4	7	2
Bnuclei	7	8	8	1
BChromatin	7	5	6	2
Nnucleoli	9	4	3	1
Mitoses	4	2	2	1
Benign	0	10	1	433
Malign	94	91	45	9

Table 3.5. *Cluster centres and cluster class composition for* k = 3

	1	2	3
Clump	7	7	3
UnifCellSize	8	5	1
UnifCellsHhape	8	5	1
MargAdhesion	7	5	1
SECSize	7	4	2
Bnuclei	7	9	1
BChromatin	7	5	2
Nnucleoli	8	4	1
Mitoses	3	2	1
Benign	0	10	434
Malign	123	102	14

evenly spread through the other clusters. This heterogeneity is also highlighted if the data are subjected to a MDS (Figure 3.15). The MDS plot shows that the malignant cases are much more widely spread out along the first (x) axis than the benign cases, although there are a few benign outliers and a small cluster at the upper right

This unsupervised classification has almost the same accuracy as the supervised methods used in Chapter 5. The fact that an unsupervised method can separate the classes, even though no class information was included in the analysis, suggests that there is a strong structure to the data that is created by the

Table 3.6. *Cluster centres and cluster class composition for* k = 2

	1	2
Clump	3	7
UnifCellSize	1	7
UnifCellsHhape	1	7
MargAdhesion	1	6
SECSize	2	5
Bnuclei	1	8
BChromatin	2	6
Nnucleoli	1	6
Mitoses	1	3
Benign	435	9
Malign	18	221

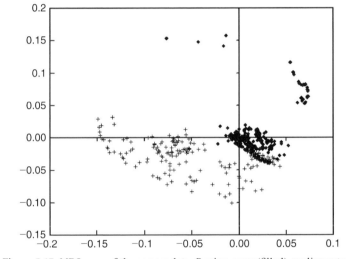

Figure 3.15 MDS map of the cancer data. Benign cases (filled), malignant cases (cross).

major differences in the class values across the variables used in the analysis. In many analyses it is likely that class labels would not be available; if they were, a supervised classification analysis would normally be more appropriate. In the absence of class labels the results of the cluster analysis would have to be subjected to some post-processing. For example, the table of mean values (Table 3.6) from the *k*-means analysis of the cancer data clearly indicates the presence of two groups that are characterised by low and high values for the means of all of the variables.

4

Introduction to classification

4.1   Background

Classifying objects or, more generally, recognising patterns is not a simple task for automated procedures, particularly when the objects are of biological interest. For example, identifying species, predicting species distributions or finding gene expression patterns that predict the risk of developing a particular type of tumour are generally difficult tasks. In this book the tool responsible for the classification is called a classifier and the term encompasses a wide range of designs, some of which are described in the next chapters.

The first attempts at biological pattern recognition tended to use statistical methods, for example discriminant analysis and logistic regression, but more recently a wider range of techniques has been used, including some that have 'borrowed' ideas from biology. Although a wide range of algorithms is covered in these pages, it is impossible to be comprehensive. However, the techniques that have been included should help readers to understand the logic of other techniques.

Jain *et al.* (2000) recognised four distinct approaches to pattern recognition. The first approach, and the main theme of their paper, was statistical. These methods find decision boundaries by making use of information about the class probability distributions. The second approach is one of the simplest and relies on matching cases to class templates or exemplars. The third is little used in biology and relies on decomposing patterns into sub-patterns, which may also be broken down further. This hierarchical approach is called syntactic because of its similarity to the structure of language. For example, a sentence can be decomposed into words, which can then be further decomposed into the constituent letters. The syntactic approach is not covered in more detail in this book. The final approach recognised by Jain *et al.* (2000) uses artificial neural networks (Section 6.4). However, it is not always clear how different some neural networks are from statistical methods.

Understanding the theory underlying statistical classifiers is not easy for most biologists, and this is complicated by the need to consider multivariate rather than univariate data. In the univariate case it is possible to estimate the probability of drawing a single observation from a population of values with a known probability distribution. For example, IQ is normally distributed with a mean of 100 and a standard deviation of 15. The *z* statistic can be used to find the proportion of the population with an IQ greater or less than a specified value. For example, the probability of selecting, at random, a person with an IQ $\geq$ 130 is 2.28%. Similarly, in a multivariate classification problem, it is possible to estimate the probability that a vector $\mathbf{x}$ (a series of observations from different variables) was drawn from a particular class as long as the class-conditional probability function, $p(\mathbf{x}|\text{class}_i)$, is known. Under the assumption of known class probability density functions it can be shown that the best classifier is a Baye's decision rule. This is a method that calculates the probability of drawing a particular vector from a class. Indeed the error from a Baye's rule is the minimum possible error rate for a particular data set that cannot be decreased by any other classifier and thereby provides a lower boundary against which other classifiers can be judged. Although naïve Baye's classifiers (Section 5.2) are known to work well, there are few real examples where class-conditional probability distributions are known. Instead they have to be estimated (learned) from the training data. This means that there will be uncertainty about the relevant parameters (means, standard deviations, etc.) that make it impossible to obtain the true class-conditional probability distributions. Because the parameter values have to be estimated from the training data their effectiveness is dependent on factors such as the size and composition of the training data. This also makes classifiers susceptible to the 'curse of dimensionality'.

The curse of dimensionality is a function of the ratio of training cases to class predictor variables. If there are too many predictors the reliability of the parameter estimates declines. In addition, providing more predictors may, in reality, reduce the classifier's performance. This is known as Watanabe's (1985) 'ugly duckling' theorem, which states that adding sufficient irrelevant predictors can sometimes make cases from different classes more similar and hence degrade performance. This is also seen in the comparison between binary similarity measures, some of which (e.g. the simple matching coefficient) include joint absences in their measure of similarity. The lesson from these related problems is that care should be taken to ensure that the number of potential predictors should be minimised and optimised. In the machine learning community this reduction in the number of predictors is known as feature selection, although many biologists will only be familiar with the stepwise variable selection algorithms that are built into most commercial statistical packages.

Using judgement, rather than automated procedures, to select predictors should be encouraged since it demands careful consideration of the problem. For example, although variable selection is generally based on statistical criteria, common sense has a part to play. If two models have similar statistical validity or predictive accuracy, but one includes variables that are expensive or time consuming to collect, it should be rejected in favour of the less-expensive model. Huberty (1994) suggested three variable screening techniques including logical screening. His approach uses theoretical, reliability and practical grounds to screen variables. Huberty suggests using subject-specific knowledge to find variables that may have some theoretical link with the classes. He also thinks that it is wise to take account of data reliability and the practical problems of obtaining data; this includes cost (time or financial) factors. Statistical screening is Huberty's second technique. This uses statistical tests to identify variables whose values differ significantly between groups. Huberty suggests applying a relaxed criterion, which only rejects those variables that are most likely to be 'noise' (e.g. $F < 1.0$ or $t < 1.0$). In addition, inter-predictor correlations should be examined to find those variables that are 'highly correlated'. Redundant variables should be removed. Hand (1997), in a very useful review of methods, also covers approaches to variable selection when building classifiers.

Jain *et al.* (2000) point out the need to separate 'feature selection' from 'feature extraction'. The first refers to algorithms that select a subset of predictors from a larger list (e.g. Huberty's second technique and stepwise variable selection algorithms). Unfortunately only the computationally expensive exhaustive search methods, which try all predictor combinations, are guaranteed to find the optimal selection of predictors. As the number of predictors increases variable selection becomes difficult, even on modern fast computers. Instead heuristic search strategies are used that may find a different subset of predictors depending on, for example, the direction of the search (growing or reducing the predictors). Feature extraction, which is the third of Huberty's (1994) criteria, creates a smaller set of new variables from those available. Two of the more common feature extraction techniques are PCA (Section 2.5.2) and MDS (Section 2.6.2). Both methods produce a smaller set of derived variables but they differ fundamentally in the criteria used. Because a method, such as PCA, also has the advantage of removing any predictor collinearity it can serve a dual purpose. Variable selection is discussed again in Section 4.6.

4.2   Black-box classifiers

Imagine a machine that could reliably identify species of arthropod, perhaps restricted to one group such as the Lepidoptera. This would be a very powerful survey tool and, as long as it was accurate, we might not be too concerned with the mechanics of the identification process and a 'black box' would be acceptable. Given our poor taxonomic knowledge for many arthropod groups it would also be helpful if the machine recognised 'new' species, even if it could not name them. There have been several attempts to produce automatic species identification systems. For example, Boddy *et al.* (2000) and Wilkins *et al.* (2001) used artificial neural networks to identify phytoplankton, while Do *et al.* (1999) investigated automated systems for spider recognition. Gaston and Neil (2004), in a review of the potential for automated species identification systems, concluded that progress was encouraging and that such approaches had great potential benefits.

May (1998) and Riordan (1998) are other examples where a black-box approach to identification is acceptable. The corncrake *Crex crex* is globally threatened and Britain's migrant population has a much reduced distribution, breeding mainly in less intensively farmed western isles such as Coll and Tiree. It is not an easy bird to census visually but the male's distinctive call enables population estimates to be made. In his work May investigated if it was possible to recognise individuals from their calls. If this is possible we may be able to improve our understanding of corncrake ecology and ensure that censuses are unbiased. Despite statistical evidence for significant variation, the classifiers (artificial neural networks) were robust enough to cope with between-night variation. May suggested that it may be possible to implement a complete system in hardware, a real black box that could extract key features from a call in real time and pass them to a neural network for immediate identification. Similarly, Riordan (1998) addressed the problem of recognising individual large carnivores from their signs, footprints in his example. The problem addressed by Riordan was can we correctly assign footprints to individuals when there is no information about the individuals, or even how many individuals there are? Although the aim was to develop a technique that can be used in the field with unknown animals, his preliminary study used known animals so that the performance of the classifiers could be validated. Autoclass (a Bayesian mixture-modelling approach, Section 3.3.3) was able to discriminate successfully between the prints from different animals and it correctly identified the number of animals. Both of these systems, although lacking explanatory power, could be of great biological value because of their predictive power.

Now imagine a different classifier that can tell, from a plasma sample, which patients are susceptible to particular types of cancer. While this prognosis may be of immediate benefit (if only to an insurance company) it would be frustrating if no information was provided on how the conclusion was reached. Knowing which factors were important for each cancer could suggest research avenues leading to the development of prophylactics or treatments. Similarly, it would be useful if a classifier was able to pick out those species most at threat from extinction. In the short term, given the current level of threat, it is probably acceptable to have a classifier that predicts without explanation, but in the medium term we would want to understand the combination of characteristics which increase extinction proneness.

The lesson from these examples is that we need to decide if interpretability is important when deciding which classification or prediction algorithms are appropriate for a particular problem. Even then it should be recognised that interpretability is a relative term. For example, decision trees produce rules that relatively untrained users can understand while the same cannot be said for the output from a logistic regression or an artificial neural network. The need to be able to communicate research findings to an educated, but non-subject-specialist audience should not be underestimated.

4.3   Nature of a classifier

Most supervised learning methods used by classifiers are inductive, i.e. they extract general patterns from data. Usually these patterns are extracted from a subset of cases known as the training data. It is generally advisable to test the predictor on a new data set called the test or validation data (see Chapter 7). If it performs well with novel data it is possible to have some confidence in the classifier's future use.

It is important to understand that the class separation and identification achieved by all classifiers is constrained by the application of some algorithm to the data. For example, many statistical methods assume that classes can be separated by a linear function. This means that they will suffer if the boundaries between the classes are non-linear. The linear nature of many classifiers is well illustrated by linear discriminant analysis, which assigns class membership following the application of some threshold to a discriminant score calculated from $\Sigma b_i x_i$, where x_i are the predictor variables and b_i are the weights of each predictor. The problem reduces to one of estimating the values of the coefficients (b_i) using a maximum-likelihood procedure that depends on an assumed probability density function. Because the values of these coefficients are unknown, but presumed to be fixed, the emphasis is on the structure of the separation rule rather than the individual cases. Statistical classifiers usually provide confidence intervals for the parameter estimates, but these are conditional on having specified the appropriate statistical model and the classification accuracy of a technique such as logistic regression is largely independent of the goodness of fit (Hosmer and Lemeshow, 1989). Part of the problem is that, for all methods, classification accuracy is sensitive to the group sizes (prevalence), and cases are more likely to be assigned to the largest group. As the prevalence declines it becomes increasingly difficult to find rules that predict the minority class. Thus, the criteria by which statistical classifiers are usually judged relate to the statistical model rather than the classification accuracy. This represents a fundamental difference between traditional statistical methods and the newer machine learning methods, where the classifier's accuracy is usually central to the assessment of a classifier's value.

There is some growing support for the need to rethink our approaches to the application of classifiers to biological problems. In particular the emphasis should move away from statistical concerns, such as the goodness of fit, to more pragmatic issues (Table 4.1).

Altman and Royston (2000) summarised this succinctly when they noted that 'usefulness is determined by how well a model works in practice, not by how many 0s there are in associated p values'. They also point out that a statistically valid model may be clinically invalid (too weak) and vice versa. For example, a model could be clinically valid but fail statistically because it is biased or has a poor goodness of fit. These, plus other concerns, lead to the general conclusion that an ideal classifier would be accurate, with utility and an ability to handle costs. Unfortunately all of these characteristics are rather vague and open to different interpretations.

Accuracy can be defined as 'faithful measurement of the truth'. However, this assumes that there is a truth against which predictions can be assessed.

Table 4.1. *A comparison of statistical and pragmatic issues that should be considered during classifier development (based on Table 1 in Hosking et al., 1997)*

Statistical issues	Pragmatic issues
Model specification	Model accuracy
Parameter estimation	Generalisability
Diagnostic checks	Model complexity
Model comparisons	Cost

The robustness of the truth or gold standard against which classifier performance is judged is an important, and often overlooked, issue. While true classes are unambiguous in some circumstances, e.g. forged versus valid bank notes, there are others in which the distinction between classes is less clear. For example, in species distribution modelling classifiers are used to predict the distribution of species, which are almost always rare or endangered. When a species population is below its carrying capacity there may be many locations that are suitable but currently vacant. A simple comparison of a classifier's predictions against this current distribution is likely to result in a reduced accuracy. It is almost impossible to judge the true quality of this classifier unless, and until, the population expands and individuals occupy the locations predicted by the classifier. It is important, in situations like this, to think carefully about how accuracy should be measured (Fielding, 1999b, 2002; Fielding and Bell, 1997).

Ripley (1996) suggests that a classifier should be capable of reporting three outcomes when presented with an object whose class is unknown:

1.   make a class prediction (usual outcome);
2.   identify the case as not belonging to a target class (outlier);
3.   inform the user that the object cannot be identified (reject).

Unfortunately most biological classifiers fail to make use of the second and third outcomes, often compromising their performance. As Ripley (1996) explains, if the classifier suggests that the case is too hard to classify it could be passed to another classifier, possibly a human, for further processing.

A dictionary definition of utility is that it is a measure of the total benefit or disadvantage to each of a set of alternative courses of action. This is a useful definition because it suggests that the utility of a classifier could be assessed from a list of its advantages/disadvantages. This would then allow comparisons to be made between classifiers. But, what are the factors, apart from accuracy, that may contribute to the advantages and disadvantages of a classifier? Four possible criteria are: speed of computation; comprehensibility of output; availability and complexity of software; and, importantly, acceptability (by peers). It is also important to bear in mind what Einstein is supposed to have said about explanations: 'The best explanation is as simple as possible, but no simpler.'

The advantages and disadvantages by which a classifier's utility is judged can be set into a cost framework. Although it is impossible to construct cost-free classifiers, it is possible to forget that there are costs. For example, failure to impose a misclassification cost structure implies that all misclassifications carry the same costs. It is often thought that costs are largely restricted to machine learning methods but it is possible to incorporate them into standard statistical methods by adjustments to the significance level, which will alter the probability of type I and II errors. As Fisher stated in 1925, 'No scientific worker has a fixed level of significance from year to year, and in all circumstances, he rejects hypotheses; he rather gives his mind to each particular case in the light of his evidence and his ideas.' Unfortunately adjustments to the significance level are fraught with difficulties since it is a component of the power of a test. However, there is much more to classifier costs than misclassification. Four categories of cost apply to all classifiers. First, there are costs associated with the predictors (data), which may be complex if some costs are shared between predictors (Turney, 1995). These costs would be considered during the classifier's development (e.g. Schiffers, 1997; Turney, 1995). Second, there are computational costs, which include the time spent pre-processing the data, learning how to use the classifier and the computer resources that are needed to run the classifier (a measure of the utility). Third are the costs associated with the misclassified cases. Finally, there are costs related to the acceptability of a method to our peers. When we write up our work it must go through the review process and we all have conservative colleagues!

Accuracy, costs and, by implication, utility are covered in much greater detail in Chapter 7.

4.4   No-free-lunch

Which is the best classifier? It is possible to phrase this question within two contexts. In the first the comparison would be between classifiers with different designs while the second compares different instances of one classifier, for example a logistic regression with different predictor sets.

Although this is an obvious question to ask prior to developing a classifier, it is an impossible one to answer. Wolpert and Macready's (1995) no-free-lunch (NFL) theorem is a proof that there is no 'best' algorithm over all possible classification problems. Wolpert and Macready (1995) say that 'all algorithms that search for an extremum of a cost function perform exactly the same, when averaged over all possible cost functions'. This theorem implies that although one classifier may outperform another on problem A, it is possible that the ranking would be reversed for problem B. Indeed the NFL theorem shows that it is impossible, in the absence of prior domain knowledge, to choose between two algorithms based on their previous behaviour. The original and additional papers on this topic can be obtained from http://www.no-free-lunch.org.

The existence of the NFL theorem means that other factors, such as size of the training set, missing values and probability distributions, are likely to be more important guides to the choice of classifier algorithm. It also suggests that algorithm comparisons should be treated with caution, or at least with a recognition that the algorithm rankings are probably only applicable to the specific set of data tested. Approaches to the comparison of classifiers are outlined in Section 7.9.

4.5   Bias and variance

The classifier is developed using a set of data known as the training data. It is important to understand that the role of the training data is not to produce a classifier that is capable of producing exact representations of themselves, but rather to build a general model of the relationship between the classes and the predictors. The ability to generalise is influenced by the classifier's complexity because, in general, classifiers with either too few, *or* too many, parameters may perform poorly with new data. This means that the classifier's complexity must be optimised. This difficult trade-off can be informed by taking account of the classifier's bias and variance. A classifier that is too simple may have a large bias while one with too much flexibility could have a high variance.

Bias is a measure of the classifier's accuracy, i.e. the closeness of the class predictions to the reality. Low bias implies high accuracy and is, therefore, a desirable property. Variance is a measure of precision or repeatability. If the variance is high, accuracy will change markedly between different training sets. It is difficult to have confidence in the future performance of a classifier with high variance because the current accuracy may not be repeated with different data. Consequently, a classifier with low variance is also desirable.

Although an ideal classifier would have both low bias and low variance there is an unfortunate trade-off such that one increases as the other declines. This is because low bias depends on an ability to adapt to differences in training sets, which is only possible if there are many parameters. Unfortunately a classifier with many parameters is also likely to have a high variance. Friedman (1997) provides a detailed background to the bias–variance trade-off and Duda *et al.* (2001) have a nice example (Figure 9.4, p. 467) which uses linear and quadratic regression to illustrate the bias–variance trade-off. This trade-off is reflected in the different relationships between training and testing error and classifier complexity. As the classifier complexity increases the errors within the training data should decline until some minimum is reached. However, although testing error will show an initial, parallel, decline with increasing classifier complexity it will begin to increase as the classifier passes its optimum complexity. This trend has to be incorporated into the design of decision trees and artificial neural networks to avoid developing classifiers that are sub-optimal for new data (Chapter 6).

4.6   Variable (feature) selection

4.6.1   Background

It is clear that careful selection of predictors could have a significant impact on classifier performance. A range of methods that have been used to select the best predictors are outlined in this section.

Because one of the main difficulties involved in creating effective classifiers is predictor or feature selection, it is worth spending time on this part of a classifier's design. Refining the predictors, along with their measurement, is likely to yield bigger performance gains than making the classifier more complex. The aim is to select a small series of predictors that produce accurate predictions at minimum cost. This is partly related to a heuristic (rule of thumb) that is common throughout science which states that whenever there are competing explanations we should always choose the simplest, i.e. we should attempt to select the most parsimonious solution. However, it is important to remember Einstein's alleged comment that models should be as simple as possible but no simpler. Unfortunately choosing an optimum set of predictors to simplify a model is not always easy.

Mac Nally (2000) listed four reasons why simple models should be sought. Firstly, there is a need to avoid over-fitting the model, i.e. modelling the noise in the data which will degrade the model's performance with future data. Secondly, future performance is generally lessened when there are too many predictors. Thirdly, simple models are thought to provide a better insight into causality. Finally, reducing the number of predictors reduces the economic cost of current and future data collection. However, as Burnham and Anderson (2004) noted there is a conflict between the need to produce a parsimonious model, that does not model noise, and the need to develop a model that is capable of representing the complexity within the data, i.e. there is a requirement to balance the classifier's bias against its variance.

It is important to realise that selection of variables always involves compromises but the selections should be driven primarily by domain-specific knowledge. Unfortunately the compromises are generally the consequences of cost and availability. As Fogarty said, in the context of genetic algorithms, 'the way that you represent the problem space embodies knowledge about a problem'. This means that there is a potential danger in knowledge-poor disciplines such as ecology, where there may be a temptation to use the same variables as other studies, without the recognition that their previous inclusion was almost certainly a result of pragmatism (what was available or could be easily recorded). In addition, if a large number of irrelevant predictors are used Watanabe's (1985) 'ugly duckling' theorem will apply. The irrelevant predictors, which carry no information about class membership, will tend to make cases from different classes more similar and hence degrade a classifier's performance, whilst also increasing the variance. Therefore, prior to their inclusion in the classifier, it is generally useful to subject potential predictors to a considerable amount of exploratory data analysis (EDA) and some pre-processing (Chapter 2), possibly reducing their dimensionality. However, it can be dangerous to rely on the univariate characteristics of a predictor because its relationship with other predictors may be more important than its independent effect.

Burnham and Anderson's (2004) review of the use of the Akaike (AIC) and Bayesian information criteria (BIC) in model selection is well worth reading but it is important to understand that their views are predicated on the superiority of the ITMC approach. The ITMC approach assumes that there is a relatively small, a priori, set of models developed that are founded on current scientific understanding. As such their approach should not be viewed as a 'blind' search for the best model from all possible models; indeed they are critical of such approaches.

4.6.2   *Variable selection methods*

Signal-to-noise ratio

One guide to the appropriate predictors is their variability within the classes relative to the differences between the classes, i.e. their signal-to-noise ratios. For example, consider two predictors which have means of 100 (class A), 110 (class B) and 100 (class A), 105 (class B) for two classes. The difference in the means suggests that the first predictor should be better because the difference between the means is twice as large. However, if the pooled standard deviations were 20.0 and 5.0 it is likely that the second predictor would be the better predictor. In this respect it is similar to the concept of statistical power. The ability to find a significant difference between two or more statistical populations is related to the effect size (the degree of difference) and the experimental error (within-population variability). This is reflected in the usual calculations for a test statistic such as t or F, which are essentially ratios of between-population differences divided by the pooled within-population variability. For example, in microarray studies there are often a large number of gene expression ratios. Many of these ratios will have little variance across the classes and will contribute nothing to discriminating between them.

EDA methods can be used to identify which genes can be excluded with little information loss.

Sequential selection methods

As the number of predictor variables rises so does the number of possible models, especially if interactions and quadratic (squared) terms are also included. There are a number of automated techniques available for deciding which variables to include in a model, for example forward and backward selection. In forward selection the first model has only one predictor (the 'best' as identified by measures such as R^2 values), the second model has two predictors, the third three, etc. The process of adding variables continues until adding more variables does not lead to a significant increase in, for example, the model R^2 value. Backward selection works in reverse since the first model includes all of the variables. These are then removed one by one until there is a significant decrease in the fit of the model. Unfortunately these two methods may generate different 'best' models.

If the number of predictor variables is small a best subsets approach can be used which fits models using all possible combinations of the predictor variables. The number of possible models is 2^p; for example, if $p = 8$ the number of different models is $2^8 = 256$. As an example, assume there are three predictors a, b and c; using a best subsets approach the following eight (2^3) models would be fitted (the constant term has been left out for clarity):

The first three are simple bivariate models

$y = a$
$y = b$
$y = c$

The next three are bivariate models

$y = a \mid b$
$y = a + c$
$y = b + c$
$y = a + b + c$
($y =$ constant is the eighth possible model)

Using appropriate diagnostic statistics the best model could then be selected. It is quite likely that the full model ($y = a + b + c$) will have the best fit (e.g. largest R^2 value), but is this R^2 much larger than any of the one- or two-predictor models? If it is not perhaps the principle of parsimony should be applied and the best one- or two-predictor model selected.

One of the many difficulties with stepwise predictor selection approaches is that the current structure of the model restricts the next step of the analysis if variables are fixed once added or removed from the model. Some analyses allow all variables, irrespective of their current status, to be considered at each step. This can mean that a variable added at an earlier stage of a forward selection procedure may be removed and replaced by a different variable at a later stage and vice versa for backward selection. Thus, it is possible to have a model development proceeding as follows (a to e are predictor variables):

$$y = d$$
$$y = d + a$$
$$y = d + a + c$$
$$y = a + c + b + e, \text{ etc.}$$

Dougherty (2001), within the context of microarray data, explains how adding variables in a stepwise fashion can reduce the prediction error but simultaneously increase the design error. A design error is the difference between the minimum possible error (Baye's error) and that from the current model. The error from any classifier can never be less than the Baye's error, except as a consequence of sampling error in small samples, but the difference is expected to decline as the sample size increases. This may not happen if there are design errors resulting from stepwise selection algorithms.

Gene expression data

Microarray experiments typically generate data that have a very large predictors:cases ratio. For example, it is not uncommon to find data sets with expression data from 5000 to 10 000 genes obtained from less than 100 cases. If these data are going to be used with classifiers it is essential that the number of genes is reduced. Fortunately, many genes have almost constant expression levels across the samples, enabling them to be removed with very little loss of information. Dudoit *et al.* (2002) used the ratio of between-class to within-class sums of squares and selected those genes with the largest ratios. However, even after their removal the number of genes will still be excessive and a variable selection, or dimension reduction, algorithm must be employed. A PCA of the gene expression levels is often used to obtain a smaller set of orthogonal predictors (e.g. Xiong *et al.*, 2000). Bo and Jonassen (2002) raised the possibility that selection algorithms, which consider only single genes, will miss sets of genes which, in combination, would enable good class separation. Figure 5.2 is an example where two variables provide a much better class separation than either variable by itself. Bo and Jonassen (2002) suggested that this was the reason why

Xiong *et al.* (2000) achieved better accuracy using the first seven principal components rather than the 'best' 42 genes. Bo and Jonassen's (2002) method scores pairs of genes, using a simple discriminant function. The genes forming the best pair are removed before searching for the next best pair. This helps to ensure that uninformative genes are not piggy-backing on one good gene. They also describe a computationally less intensive algorithm that ranks genes by their *t*-statistics and then finds pairs whose combined *t*-statistics are the largest. In many respects this is similar to the variable selection routines suggested by Huberty (1994; Section 5.3.2), but with an extension to using pairs of variables. Lee *et al.* (2005) compared the performance of many classifiers across seven microarray datasets and one of their main conclusions was that predictor selection was one of the most important factors that influenced the accuracy of the classifiers. It is probably sensible to accept that there is no method which guarantees to find the best subset of predictors. Indeed, as shown in the genetic algorithm examples (Chapter 6), there may be a range of 'best' predictor subsets that produce classifiers with the same accuracy.

4.6.3   *Ranking the importance of predictors*

In Section 4.2 the differences between black-box (predictive) and explanatory models were discussed. These differences become very important when automated variable selection is being used. The main difficulty arises from the inter-predictor correlations. Unless all of the predictors are orthogonal (uncorrelated), it is unlikely that any variable selection routine will select out the correct causal predictors, even if the selection produced a simple and accurate classifier.

Identifying the optimum suite of predictors is only possible if all possible models are tested. Even then, procedures are needed to identify the 'best' of the resulting 2^p models and also estimating the independent effects of each predictor. Measures such as the AIC and BIC are often used to identify the best model by trading off model fit against model complexity (number of predictors). The use of information criteria is discussed further in Section 5.6.3 and Burnham and Anderson (2004) review much of the theoretical foundations for these methods. However, it is important to distinguish between an efficient classifier, that has a statistically valid set of predictors, and a classifier that includes the predictors which have a causal relationship with the class.

While this means that variable and model selection algorithms are suitable for the generation of parsimonious models, the resultant models should not be interpreted as causal. If the independent contributions by the predictors are required an alternative approach, such as hierarchical partitioning, is needed (e.g. Chevan and Sutherland, 1991; Mac Nally, 2000). However, it is important to realise that this approach is not a variable selection algorithm: rather it contributes to an explanation of the relationships between the classes and the predictors. Hierarchical partitioning can be used with a generalised linear model such as logistic regression and it works by examining classifiers with all possible predictor combinations and then averaging a predictor's influence over all classifiers that include it. This is achieved by variance partitioning. The result is an estimate of the total independent effect of each predictor, which allows variables to be identified that have spurious significant associations with the classes. Such variables would have a large association but little independent effect, i.e. their association arises because of their relationships with other important predictors. The explanatory power of each predictor is split into two components: I is the independent effect and J is the joint effect (i.e. in conjunction with other predictors). In some respects this is similar to the communality measure in a factor analysis.

4.7   Multiple classifiers

4.7.1   Background

It is well known that if one estimated a population mean from different random samples it is unlikely that the sample means would be identical, although all would be unbiased estimates of the population mean. The same is true with classifiers: the accuracy of a classifier will change if a different random sample of training cases is used. This property can be exploited by running many instances of the same classifier on resampled data to obtain a better estimate of a classifier's accuracy. It is assumed that the additional computational load will be balanced by an improved performance. If classifier predictions can be combined the prediction for a single case would not be derived from one classifier; instead some method must be found for using the information from a suite of classifiers. There is a variety of techniques that pool together the predictions from multiple classifiers. These combinations of classifiers are also known as ensembles and, typically, they work by using a majority vote. There are two broad classes of classifier ensembles: single and mixed algorithm. Single algorithm ensembles are the most common and they alter the classifier parameters or training set characteristics by techniques such as boosting and bagging (next section). The mixed algorithm ensembles combine the predictions from a range of algorithms and thereby exploit any differences in the algorithmic biases.

4.7.2   Boosting and bagging

Boosting and bagging are two methods for voting classification algorithms that differ in the rules used to obtain the multiple samples. In both cases the same classifier is used over a large number of training sets which are obtained by resampling the training data. The bagging algorithms do not use previous results to refine the training sets, while boosting algorithms refine the training set using information from earlier classifiers. Bagging, or bootstrap aggregation, uses normal bootstrap methods to obtain a large number of samples that are used to train the classifier. A final classifier uses a simple majority vote, over all of the classifiers, to estimate the classes for the cases.

Friedman *et al.* (2000) define boosting as 'a way of combining the performance of many "weak" classifiers to produce a "powerful committee"'. One form of boosting, AdaBoost (adaptive boosting), is said to be one of the best classifiers, partly because it seems to be resistant to over-fitting and it is capable of simultaneously reducing both bias and variance (Friedman *et al.*, 2000). Boosting was developed originally by Schapire (1990) as a way of improving classifier performance. In its original form a weak learner (a classifier that outperforms chance) was improved by creating two extra training sets. These new training sets were not random samples. Half of the cases in the first of these additional sets would have been misclassified by the original classifier. The second of the additional training sets contains cases on which the first two classifiers disagreed. The final class prediction for each case is a majority vote over the three classifiers. This approach was extended to create the AdaBoost algorithm (Freund and Schapire, 1996). The AdaBoost algorithm changes case weights based on the results of earlier classifiers so that the weight of misclassified cases is half of the original training set weights while correctly classified cases make up the other half. The aim of this approach is to 'boost' the importance of incorrectly classified cases so that future classifiers will attempt to correct the errors. Bauer and Kohavi (1999) compared a range of boosting and bagging algorithms and concluded that, although boosting algorithms were generally better, there were some problems with boosting algorithms such as inappropriate weighting of noise and outliers. There have been a range of subsequent modifications including Dettling's (2004) hybrid boosting and bagging algorithm, called Bagboosting. Although no mathematical proof is available, simulation studies, using gene array data, suggest that it combines advantages from both to produce a prediction tool with lower bias and variance. The combination uses the aggregated output from several base classifiers (which use resampled data) at each iteration of the boosting algorithm.

4.7.3   Combining different classifiers

The rationale behind combining predictions from different classifier algorithms is that the combinations may dilute the different biases of the classifiers. There are three main approaches to combining classifiers, depending on the measurement level of the outputs. If only predicted class labels are available the combination usually uses a majority vote. For example, if there are five classifiers a case will be labelled with a class that receives at least three votes. Slightly more information is available if the rank order of the cases is known, i.e. cases are ordered by decreasing likelihood of class membership. In principle, the most information is provided if the actual classifier scores are used. However, it is normally necessary to normalise the scores so that they share a common measurement scale. Despite the general acceptance of the need for normalisation it has been suggested that this can lead to some undesirable side-effects (Altinçay and Demirekler, 2003).

4.8   Why do classifiers fail?

Despite one's best efforts it should not be too surprising if the classifier does not perform well, particularly with new data. Understanding the potential causes of poor performance can be a useful guide to possible alterations that may improve performance. Classifiers fail to make sufficiently accurate predictions in a number of circumstances.

1. The form of the classifier is too complex and over-fits the data. This tends to arise when the parameter:cases ratio exceeds some desirable limit and the classifier begins to fit the random noise in the training data. This will lead to poor generalisation. This is why simple models often outperform complex models on novel data.
2. The form of the classifier is too simple or has an inappropriate structure. For example, classes may not be linearly separable or important predictors have been excluded (e.g. Conroy *et al.*, 1995). This will reduce accuracy.
3. If some of the training class labels are incorrect or 'fuzzy' there will be problems. Most classifiers assume that class membership in the training data is known without error. Obviously if class definitions are ambiguous, it becomes more difficult to apply a classification procedure, and any measure of accuracy is likely to be compromised. Although the assumption of known class memberships is reasonable for discrete classes such as gender or taxa, it is questionable in other situations, for example when an individual is classed as cancer-prone or cancer-free.

If cases are initially mislabelled this is likely to affect the number of prediction errors. More importantly mislabelled cases can influence the structure of the classifier, leading to bias or classifier degradation. For example, a misclassified case is likely to be an outlier for some predictors, but its influence will depend on the classifier. In a discriminant analysis outliers may have large effects because of their contribution to the covariance matrix. Conversely, in decision trees their influence on the classification rules may be trivial because they are assigned to their own branch (Bell, 1999).

4. Training cases may be unrepresentative. If they are this leads to bias and poor performance when the classifier is applied to new cases. Careful sampling designs should avoid this problem but such bias may be unavoidable if there is, for example, significant unrecognised regional and temporal variability.

5. Unequal class sizes – most classifiers will favour the most common class. Many classifiers have options to help avoid this by adjusting the class prior probabilities to values that do not represent the class proportions in the training data. Alternatively, the predictions can be post-processed by adjusting the decision threshold that is used to allocate cases to classes (Chapter 7).

4.9   Generalisation

A general theme throughout this chapter has been that classifiers should be judged by their future performance. This is because there is little to be gained if a classifier's predictive ability is restricted to the data that were used to generate it. Classifiers need to be able to work with new data, i.e. their performance should be general rather than tuned to the training data. Because classifier training is effectively learning from examples the generalisation concept can be illustrated using an educational metaphor. Most readers will have some experience of multiple choice questions (MCQs) during their education. If formative MCQs (used for education/training rather than formal assessment) were used the hope of the educator was that the student would learn some general biological principles rather than the correct answers to each question. In a summative assessment (the marks count towards an award) novel questions would have been used. A student who did well on the formative questions, but poorly on the summative questions, would not have generalised their knowledge. It is probable they attempted to learn the match between specific questions and answers, rather than gain the more general knowledge being tested. This is the same problem faced by classifier designers: they want a classifier that 'learns' the general features of the training ('formative') cases so that it will cope well with the real test of novel ('summative') cases. Assessing performance is considered in greater detail in Chapter 7.

4.10   Types of classifier

Classifier descriptions and example analyses are split across the next two chapters. In Chapter 5 the 'traditional' statistical methods, and their derivatives, are described. Most of the chapter is concerned with discriminant analysis and logistic regression. Chapter 6 describes a diverse set of classifiers that are based on different paradigms. However, the main focus is on decision trees and artificial neural networks.

5

Classification algorithms 1

5.1   Background

This chapter focuses on what might be considered the 'traditional' statistical approaches to class prediction, in particular general and generalised linear models (GLMs) such as discriminant analysis and logistic regression. It also describes a more recent, related, method called generalised additive modelling (GAM).

The role of a statistical classifier is to identify which class is the most probable, given the available information and certain assumptions about the model structure and the probability distributions. The available information is derived from the values of the predictor variables, while the assumptions depend on the approach.

A typical statistical classifier or model aims to describe the relationship between the class and the predictor. Usually, there will also be some unexplained variation (prediction errors), or noise, that we hope is caused by chance factors and not some deficiency in the model. The statistical classifier, ignoring the noise, can be summarised as class = $f(w_i x_i)$, where w_i are weights that are applied to the p predictors (x_i) to produce a weighted sum from which the class is derived. This format specifies a classifier that is linear with respect to its parameters and which can be envisaged as a plane that separates the classes in p-dimensional predictor space. The problem becomes one of identifying the appropriate values for the weights. One way of thinking about this is in terms of a recipe: changing the proportions (weights) of the ingredients will change the characteristics of the finished food. It is important that the ingredients are added in the correct proportions!

The simplest general linear models, such as those assumed by techniques like analysis of variance, take the form $y = f(L) + \varepsilon$. This model specifies that the value of y is the sum of a linear term ($f(L)$) plus some error (ε). This implies that all predictor variables within L have additive (independent) effects on the value of y. In a general linear model there is an additional important assumption that the errors are normally distributed with a constant variance for all values of y. Because of these assumptions the model coefficients or weights can be estimated using least squares methods. If the response is not normally distributed, or the relationship between the class and the predictors is non-linear, a GLM is appropriate.

GLMs are extensions of general linear models that allow for non-linearity and non-constant variance structures in the data (Hastie and Tibshirani, 1990). As with the general linear models there is an assumed linear relationship between the mean of the response variable and the predictors. However, the linear component is established, indirectly, via a link function that constrains the predicted values to fall within the range $0-1$. In addition, the GLMs can use a response variable that comes from any distribution within the exponential family of probability distributions, which includes the normal, binomial and Poisson. However, if the response variable is not normally distributed the values of the model coefficients, or weights, must be estimated using maximum likelihood, rather than least squares, techniques.

Although the GLM, $y = g(L) + \varepsilon$, has a superficial similarity to the general linear model, there are important differences. The $g(L)$ term is made up of two components, a linear term plus a link function. The link function transforms the underlying non-linear part of a model into a set of linear parameters and is normally written as g(expected value) $= L$, where L is a function that combines the predictors in a linear fashion. The form of the link function is related to the probability distribution of the response (Table 5.1).

Statistical models are usually assessed by the 'fit' between the data and the model; the 'strength' of the relationship (statistical significance) and the role of the predictors in determining the value of the response variable (finding predictors whose coefficients are not zero). There are several potential problems

Table 5.1. *Generalised linear models and their link functions*

Response probability distribution	Link function	Notes
Normal	Identity	$f(L) = g(L)$, i.e. no transformation
Binomial	Logit	Log [P(event)/P(no event)] $= f(L)$
Poisson	Log	Ln(expected) $= f(L)$

with these three measures. Firstly, classical approaches for estimating the coefficients, and hence the fit of the data, assume that the correct model has been specified. In many situations the model structure will result from subjective decisions that are at least partly driven by subject knowledge and prior expectations. Secondly, biological and statistical significance do not always coincide. A predictor whose coefficient has a very small p value may not be biologically important. Finally, if stepwise methods have been used to select the predictors it is very difficult to attach too much weight to their actual, rather than statistical, contributions.

Irrespective of the model structure there is a common confusion between explanatory and predictive models. In a predictive model only the model's accuracy is important and the structure of the model is relatively unimportant, as long as it is robust. In general, models become more robust as the number of predictors declines, and hence there is a greater tendency towards parsimony in predictive models, often using variable selection algorithms (Section 4.6). However, if a model is developed for explanatory purposes the identity and weights of the predictors is the most important part of the model because these are used to infer the nature of the relationship between, in the case of a classifier, the class and the values of the predictor variables. There are methods for dealing with these problems of identifying the unique contribution made by each predictor, for example hierarchical partitioning (Section 4.6.3), which do not appear to be used widely. The contribution made by the predictors is obviously most important in an explanatory, rather than a predictive, model. In predictive models the role of predictors is less important than the accuracy of the prediction. Consequently, the use of variable selection routines that produce a more parsimonious model are generally more acceptable in predictive models.

Finally, it is important to remember that all of these methods are supervised classification algorithms. This means that known class membership is a prerequisite for the generation of classification rules.

5.2   Naïve Bayes

A naïve Bayes classifier is a probabilistic classifier that makes use of Bayesian theory and is the optimal supervised learning method if the predictors are independent (uncorrelated), given the class. This means that, if its assumptions are met, it is guaranteed to produce the most accurate predictions. It does, therefore, place an upper limit on what a classifier can achieve. Despite the obvious over-simplification of these assumptions the naïve Bayes classifier has proved be a very effective supervised learning algorithm on real data, where the assumptions do not apply. The naïve Bayes classifier gets its name because it uses Bayesian methods in an intentionally simplistic manner to obtain class predictions. The naïvety arises from the assumptions about the independence of the predictors, which are unlikely to be valid in real data. Unless the predictors have forced orthogonality, such as principal component scores, it is normal to find some dependency (correlations) between potential predictors. In an ideal world, not only would the predictors be independent, but the parameters of the independent predictor variable probability distributions, such as means and standard deviations, would also be known. However, it is usually necessary to estimate ('learn') them from samples of data. Consequently, the data in a naïve Bayes classifier will come from unknown, but estimated, probability distributions that share some interdependency. In reality it is not even necessary to use Bayesian methods to produce these predictions because the initial Bayesian model can be rewritten in a form that is computationally more feasible using maximum likelihood techniques.

Despite these apparently important deviations from the underlying assumptions, the technique appears to work well. This is because the predictions will be accurate as long as the probability of being in the correct class is greater than that for any of the incorrect classes. In other words only an approximate solution is required that has the correct rank order for class membership probabilities. The Bayes rule assigns a case to a class (k) which has the largest posterior probability given the linear combination of predictors (x): $\text{class}_i = \max_k \{p(k|x)\}$. It is possible to frame many classifiers in the same context. For example, logistic regression uses a regression method to estimate $p(k|x)$. Other techniques, such as discriminant analysis, estimate separate class conditional probabilities ($p(x) = p(x|\text{class} = k)$). Bayesian methods are then used to estimate $p(k|x)$, so that a class identity can be assigned.

5.3   Discriminant analysis

5.3.1   Introduction

This is one of the simplest and most widely used classification methods. Despite its early widespread use in biology a number of authors, particularly during the early 1990s, questioned its validity for most analyses and suggested that logistic regression (next section) was a better alternative. However, in empirical tests discriminant analysis often emerges as one of the better classifiers.

If there is information about individuals (cases), obtained from a number of predictors, it is reasonable to ask if they can be used to define groups and/or predict the group to which an individual belongs. Discriminant analysis works by creating a new variable that is a combination of the original predictors. This is done in such a way that the differences between the predefined groups, with respect to the new variable, are maximised. The most comprehensive text dealing with all aspects of discriminant analysis is Huberty's (1994) book. If you are planning to use discriminant analysis you are strongly advised to consult it. The following section is a brief overview of discriminant analysis, which should be read in conjunction with Chapter 7.

Consider a simple two-class example. The aim is to combine (weight) the predictor scores in some way so that a single new composite variable, the discriminant score, is produced. It is possible to view this as an extreme data dimension reduction technique that compresses the p-dimensional predictors into a one-dimensional line. At the end of the process it is hoped that each class will have a normal distribution of discriminant scores but with the largest possible difference in mean scores for the classes. Indeed, the degree of overlap between the discriminant score distributions can be used as a measure of the success of the technique (Figure 5.1).

Discriminant scores are calculated by a discriminant function which has the form:

$$D = w_1Z_1 + w_2Z_2 + w_3Z_3 + \ldots w_pZ_p$$

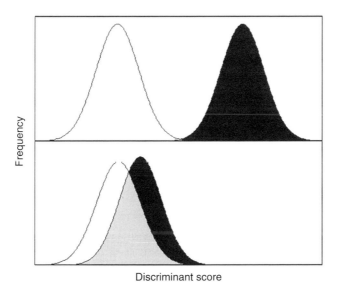

Figure 5.1 Example discriminant score distributions for two discriminant functions. In the upper example there is good discrimination with little overlap between the frequency distributions of discriminant scores for the two classes. The lower example exhibits poor discrimination and a large overlap in the frequency distributions.

where

- D = discriminant score;
- w_p = weighting (coefficient) for variable p;
- Z_p = standardised score for variable p.

Consequently a discriminant score is a weighted linear combination (sum) of the predictors. The weights are estimated to maximise the differences between class mean discriminant scores. In general, those predictors that have large differences between class means will have larger weights, whilst weights will be small when class means are similar. There are two factors that complicate the interpretation of weights. Firstly, weights will be affected by scale differences between predictors and, secondly, correlations between predictors will reduce the size of some weights. Standardising the predictors (mean of 0 and a standard deviation of 1) ensures that scale differences between predictors are eliminated. This means that absolute weights (ignore the sign) can be used to rank variables in terms of their contribution to the discriminant score, the largest weight being associated with the most powerful discriminating variable. The earlier recipe metaphor can be stretched a little more to illustrate the interpretation of weights. The quality of a finished meal is very dependent on getting the proportions of the ingredients correct. However, absolute (unstandardised) quantities are not a good guide to their contribution to the overall taste of a meal since the ingredients may have different inherent strengths (e.g. compare garlic and onion). The problems caused by correlated predictors can be overcome by using a different measure to investigate how predictors relate to the discrimination between the groups (see Section 5.3.2).

As with most other multivariate methods it is possible to use a graphical explanation problem for a simplified problem. The following example uses a simple data set, two groups and two variables. These are sepal lengths and widths for two species of *Iris*. These are the same data that were used in the EDA example in Section 2.10. If scatter graphs are plotted for scores against the two predictors Figure 5.2 is obtained.

Clearly the two species can be separated by these two variables, but there is a large amount of overlap on each axis which prevents their separation by a single variable. It is possible to construct a new axis (Figure 5.3) which passes through the two group centroids ('means'), such that the groups have little overlap on the new axis. This axis represents a new variable which is a linear combination of the predictors, i.e. a discriminant score. Because there is little overlap between the two species on this new axis a discriminant score could be used to obtain a reliable prediction of a sample's correct species.

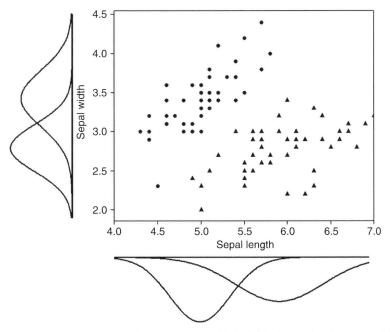

Figure 5.2 Scatter plot of two predictors with individual box plots for *I. setosa* (circles) and *I. versicolor* (triangles).

If there is more than one class it is possible to calculate more than one discriminant function, although they may not all be effective at separating the classes. The maximum number of discriminant functions is the smaller of the number of classes minus one, or the number of predictors. This means that in a two-class problem there can only be one discriminant function.

The examples below explore the simplest form of discriminant analysis. There are many other 'flavours' in use that differ with respect to the assumptions and the nature of the decision plane. Extensions to the base algorithm are briefly described in Section 5.3.3.

5.3.2   Example analyses

Three analyses are used to illustrate some of the important features of a discriminant analysis. The first two use artificial data (Appendix E) while the third is a multi-class discrimination using real data. Data set A has four predictors (a1 to a4) and two classes with 75 cases per class. The predictors are uncorrelated with each other ($p < 0.05$ for all pairwise correlations) and class means differ significantly for all predictors. This implies that all four predictors should be useful to identify the class of a case. Data set B is very similar to

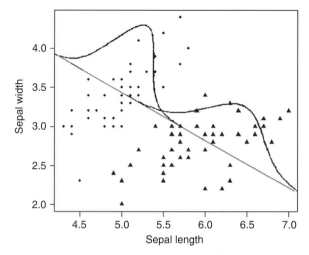

Figure 5.3 Discriminant axis and class frequency distributions for the data in Figure 5.2.

A (Table 5.2) except that variables b3 and b4 are highly correlated ($r = 0.7$); all other correlation coefficients are insignificant. If effect sizes (difference in the means divided by the standard deviation) are calculated it is possible to estimate the expected rank order for the standardised weights. In data set A the order should be a1, a3, a2, and a4, while in data set B the expected order is (b1 = b3), b2 and b4.

The third data set was used as part of study that investigated if it was possible to discriminate between the core areas of golden eagle *Aquila chrysaetos* home ranges from three regions of Scotland (Fielding and Haworth, 1995). The data consist of eight habitat variables, whose values are the amounts of each habitat

Table 5.2. *Class means and effect sizes for four predictors from two data sets. The standard deviations are common between the two data sets*

Class	a1	a2	a3	a4
1	9.8	15.2	20.7	25.1
2	11.8	17.9	24.2	29.1
Effect size	1.00	0.82	0.88	0.80
	b1	b2	b3	b4
1	9.8	15.0	20.4	25.4
2	11.8	18.1	24.4	29.1
Effect size	1.00	0.94	1.00	0.74
Common standard deviation	2.0	3.3	4.0	5.0

variable, measured as the number of four hectare blocks within a region defined as a 'core area'. The data set is described in Appendix F. This analysis is used to illustrate multi-class discrimination and a variety of predictor selection algorithms.

Discriminant analysis of two artificial data sets

Because there are two classes the maximum number of discriminant functions is one and each has an associated eigen value (λ). In these analyses the two values were 0.804 (Data set A) and 0.792 (Data set B). Larger eigen values are associated with greater class separations and they can also be used to measure the relative importance of discriminant functions in multi-class analyses. Eigen values can be converted into Wilk's lambda, a multivariate test statistic whose value ranges between zero and one. Values close to zero indicate that class means are different while values close to one indicate that the class means are not different. Wilk's lambda will be one when the means are identical. Wilk's lambda is equal to $1/(1 + \lambda)$ for a two-class problem and can be converted into a chi-square statistic so that a significance test can be applied. In these analyses the values were 0.554 (A) and 0.558 (B). The null hypothesis to be tested is that 'there is no discriminating power remaining in the variables'. If p is less than 0.05 there is evidence that predictors have some ability to discriminate between the groups. In these analyses the chi-square values (with four degrees of freedom) are 86.1 and 85.2, respectively. Since $p < 0.001$ for both analyses there is strong evidence for some discriminating power in both data sets.

Wilk's lambda can be converted into a canonical correlation coefficient from the square root of 1 − Wilk's lambda. The canonical correlation is the square root of the ratio of the between-groups sum of squares to the total sum of squares. Squared, it is the proportion of the total variability explained by differences between classes. Thus, if all of the variability in the predictors was a consequence of the group differences the canonical correlation would be one, while if none of the variability was due to group differences the canonical correlation would be zero. In these analyses the values were 0.668 (A) and 0.665 (B).

An assumption of a discriminant analysis is that there is no evidence of a difference between the covariance matrices of the classes. There are formal significance tests for this assumption (e.g. Box's M) but they are not very robust. In particular they are generally thought to be too powerful, i.e. the null hypothesis is rejected even when there are minor differences, and Box's M is also susceptible to deviations from multivariate normality (another assumption). If Box's test is applied to these data we would conclude that the covariance matrices are unequal for data set A ($M = 30.9$, $p = 0.001$) but equal for data set B ($M = 18.7$, $p = 0.052$). The inequality of the covariance matrices is more likely to be a problem when class proportions are different. Under such circumstances the pooled covariance matrix will be dominated by the larger class.

Each discriminant function can be summarised by three sets of coefficients: (1) standardised canonical discriminant function coefficients (weights); (2) correlations between discriminating variables and the standardised canonical discriminant function; and (3) unstandardised canonical discriminant function coefficients (weights). These are shown for both data sets in Table 5.3.

It is only in Table 5.3 that differences between the two data sets become apparent. All of the previous diagnostic statistics, such as Wilk's lambda, have been very similar, reflecting the similarity in the class means for the predictors. The standardised coefficients show the contribution made by each predictor to the discriminant function, after removing scale differences. As expected, for uncorrelated predictors, the weights are very similar. The slight disparity in weights reflects the differences in effect sizes combined with some minor, but insignificant, correlations between the predictors. The standardised weights for data set A are, as expected, in the same rank order as the effect sizes (Table 5.2). However, the unstandardised weights for data set B are obviously unequal, particularly for predictor b4. Using the effect sizes from Table 5.2 we should expect b1 and b3 to have the largest and similar weights. However, the b3 weight is considerably larger than that for b1. This is partly because the correlation between b3 and b4 means that b3 has some predictive power related to b4. The weight for b4 is, as expected, the smallest unstandardised weight.

Weights reflect the contribution made by a predictor, after accounting for the discrimination achieved using other predictors. Consider an extreme example

Table 5.3. *Standardised canonical discriminant function coefficients (w_s); correlations between discriminating variables and the standardised canonical discriminant function (r_{df}); and unstandardised canonical discriminant function coefficients (w_u) for the discriminant analyses of data sets A and B*

Predictor	w_s	r_{df}	w_u	Predictor	w_s	r_{df}	w_u
a1	0.598	0.486	0.260	b1	0.604	0.524	0.281
a2	0.568	0.457	0.170	b2	0.630	0.520	0.190
a3	0.596	0.479	0.144	b3	0.817	0.534	0.193
a4	0.435	0.377	0.073	b4	−0.295	0.274	−0.039
Constant			−10.85	Constant			−9.48

of two perfectly correlated predictors x and y. If x has already been used to discriminate between the classes y cannot provide any extra discrimination (even though on its own it is just as good as variable x). Recall that predictor b4 is highly correlated with b3 ($r = 0.7$). Because b4 is correlated with b3 it provides little additional information about the class differences, once b3 has been taken into account. This is reflected in its low weight. Because it is common to have some interdependency between predictors, such as that between b3 and b4, it is important to bear this in mind when interpreting the discriminant function. The low weight for b4 does not mean that its values do not differ between the classes, rather it reflects the small quantity of additional class separation information when combined with b3.

A more robust interpretation on the class differences can be obtained from the correlations between the predictors and the standardised canonical discriminant function (r_{df}). These correlations, or structure coefficients, are simple Pearson correlations between the discriminant scores and the original predictor values. Hence, some of the weight reductions cased by inter-predictor correlations, are less apparent. In this respect it is very similar to interpreting the contribution made by each variable to a principal component (Chapter 2).

The main problem with standardised coefficients is that predictor scores must be standardised before the function can be applied to new data. One solution is to obtain unstandardised coefficients, but note that it is not easy to rank these unstandardised coefficients since their magnitudes are related to the scale of their associated predictor. For example, the unstandardised discriminant function for data set A is class = $-10.85 + 0.260.a1 + 0.170.a2 + 0.144.a3 + 0.073.a4$. Note how the unstandardised coefficients decrease in size as the predictor means become larger.

The discriminant function means are -0.891 for class 1 and 0.891 for class 2. Because class sizes and prior class probabilities are equal in this data set, the boundary between the classes is a score of zero. If the discriminant score is ncgativc the predicted class is one, and two if the score is positive. Normally, classes are assigned using the maximum $P(\text{Class}|\text{Score})$, the probability of the class given the discriminant score. The probability cut-off is very strict. If, in a two-class problem, $P(\text{class 1}|\text{score}) = 0.501$ and $P(\text{class 2}|\text{score}) = 0.499$ the individual would be placed into class one. It is important to bear this in mind when judging the predictive accuracy of a discriminant function. More information about the robustness of class allocations is provided by the Mahalanobis distance. This is a measure of how far a case's values differ from the average of all cases in the class. For a single predictor, it is simply the square of its z value. A large Mahalanobis distance identifies a case as having extreme values on one or more of the predictors. Thus, it measures how far a case is from the 'mean' of its group. Note that as this increases the probability of belonging to a group decreases.

When there are many cases it is impractical to examine individuals; instead an overall summary is required. This summary is usually presented as a confusion matrix which cross-tabulates actual and predicted class membership. For the two examples summarised in Table 5.4 data are presented for re-substituted and cross-tabulated predictions. The re-substituted values are obtained by applying the discriminant function to all 150 cases and this method generally provides an optimistic assessment of the classifier's accuracy. The cross-tabulated results partly overcome this by producing a prediction for each case when it has been excluded from the generation of the discriminant function. In both cases re-substituted and cross-tabulated accuracy measures are similar and there is little to choose between the two classifiers. Aspects of classifier accuracy assessment are covered in much more detail in Chapter 7.

Discriminant analysis of golden eagle data (multi-class analysis)

Three analyses are presented which illustrate, initially, the features of a multi-class discriminant analysis and, secondly, how predictor selection algorithms can be used to produce a more robust classifier. The data were used as part of project that had the ambitious aim of predicting the effect of habitat changes on golden eagle range occupancy. The initial work was

Table 5.4. *Classification statistics for classifiers A and B. The percentage of cases correctly classified is derived from the number of class one cases predicted to be class one plus the number of class two cases predicted to be class two*

Classifier	Actual class	Re-substituted predicted class		Cross-validated predicted class	
		1	2	1	2
A	1	63	12	63	12
	2	18	57	18	57
Percentage cases correctly classified		82.0%		82.0%	
B	1	62	13	61	14
	2	14	61	15	60
Percentage cases correctly classified		82.0%		80.7%	

concerned with understanding how, and if, habitat differed across regions. The data are available in Appendix F.

Because there are three classes (different regions of Scotland) it may be possible to construct more than one discriminant function. The maximum number of discriminant functions that can be obtained is the lesser of the number of classes minus one or the number of predictors. In this example there are three classes and eight predictors so the maximum number of discriminant functions is two (Table 5.5).

The function one eigen value is almost twice as large as that for function two, suggesting greater separation between the classes. The percentage of variance for the functions indicates their relative importance and is calculated from $\lambda_t/\Sigma\lambda$. Recall that Wilk's lambda is a measure of the discriminating power remaining in the variables, and that values close to zero indicate high discriminating power. Wilk's lambda ($\Pi(1/(1+\lambda_t))$) for the first function is very close to zero, suggesting the presence of significant discriminating power. The second value ($1/(1+\lambda)$) relates to the second function and is measured after removing the discriminating power associated with the first function. The chi-squared values indicate that both functions are capable of some significant discrimination. Because there are two functions there are two sets of coefficients (Table 5.6).

The predictors are quite highly correlated with each other so the interpretation of the functions uses the structure coefficients. Function one is mainly associated with the areas of wet heath, bog and steep ground. Thus, cases with a positive score on function one tend to have more wet heath and steep ground and less bog (negative correlation). Function two is mainly associated with the area of land below 200 m, between 400 and 600 m and steep slopes. The area of wet heath is also important. Thus, cases with a positive score on function two tend to have more land below 200 m, but less steep land and land between 400 and 600 m. When there are two functions the classes are separated in two-dimensional space by Thiessen polygons centred on the class centroids (Table 5.7, Figure 5.4).

Table 5.5. *Summary of discriminant functions for golden eagle data*

Function	Eigen value (λ)	Percentage of variance	Wilk's lambda	Chi-square	df	p	Canonical correlation
1	4.513	67.2	0.057	96.134	16	0.000	0.905
2	2.198	32.8	0.313	38.945	7	0.000	0.829

Table 5.6. *Standardised canonical discriminant function coefficients and structure coefficients (correlations between discriminating variables and standardised canonical discriminant functions) for both discriminant functions. The largest absolute correlation between each predictor and any discriminant function is marked with an asterisk*

Predictor	Standardised canonical discriminant function coefficients		Structure coefficients	
	1	2	1	2
POST	0.058	0.516	−0.077	0.194*
PRE	−0.134	0.027	−0.197*	−0.010
BOG	−0.201	0.849	−0.467*	0.053
CALL	0.338	0.103	0.075	0.242*
WET	0.866	−0.063	0.631*	−0.428
STEEP	0.537	0.546	0.326	−0.555*
LT200	0.668	1.535	0.198	0.784*
L4_600	−0.138	0.221	−0.037	−0.443*

Table 5.7. *Class centroids ('mean' discriminant score) for each function*

Region	Function	
	1	2
1	−3.726	−1.680
2	2.049	−1.003
3	−0.394	1.636

The group centroids in Table 5.7 show that discriminant function one separates region 1 from region 2, with region 3 in between them, while function two separates region 3 from the other two. This is best seen in a territorial map (Figure 5.4).

The territorial map (Figure 5.4) highlights how the functions separate the groups. Class membership is determined by the combination of function one and two scores. For example, a case with a score of +4.0 and −4.0 would be placed in region 2. However, before cases can be assigned to regions the boundaries must be set using class prior probabilities. In this analysis they are set to be equal, thus all are 0.333. An alternative weighting would have been to

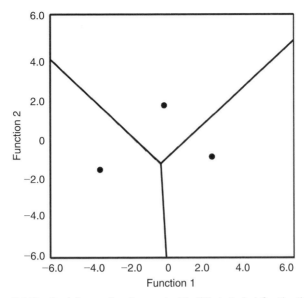

Figure 5.4 Territorial map showing centroids (filled circles) for the three areas on two discriminant functions.

Table 5.8. *Classification statistics for golden eagle range predictions*

		Predicted class		
Classifier	Actual class	1	2	3
Re-substituted	1	7	0	0
	2	0	14	2
	3	0	0	17
Percentage cases correctly classified			95.0%	
Cross-validated	1	6	0	1
	2	1	11	4
	3	0	1	16
Percentage cases correctly classified			82.5%	

set them to class sizes. For example, this would have given region 1 a prior probability of 0.175 (7/40).

The regions are very accurately predicted using the re-substitution (original data) method, only two region 2 cases are misclassified (Table 5.8). Even when using the cross-validated method, the accuracy remains good, although five region 2 cases are now misclassified. The results are shown graphically in Figure 5.5.

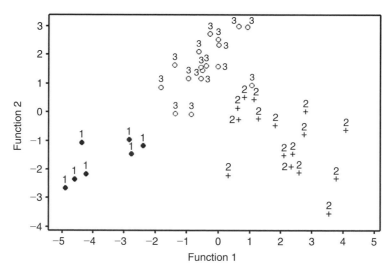

Figure 5.5 Map of class predictions; labels are the actual class. Axes are the two discriminant functions and the coordinates are the case scores on the discriminant functions.

In summary, these eight habitat variables can be used to discriminate between the core area habitats of golden eagles living in three Scottish regions. Two gradients were detected and described from the function structure coefficients. However, rather a large number of predictors (eight) were used with a relatively small number of cases (40). Such ratios tend to give very good separation. Various minimum cases:predictor ratios have been suggested in the literature, ranging between 3:1 and 5:1. The smallest class size in this analysis was seven suggesting that no more than two predictors should be used. The next analysis uses a stepwise analysis in an attempt to reduce the predictor dimensionality. This is possibly justified if the aim is a predictive classifier but if, as in this example, the aim is to understand the differences it may not be appropriate (see Section 4.6 for a critique of variable selection algorithms).

There are various stepwise options available; in this analysis a forward selection algorithm was used that selects, at each step, the predictor that minimises the overall Wilk's lambda. Details are not shown, but only three variables were selected: WET, LT200 and STEEP, giving two significant discriminant functions. Although the ideal number of predictors was two (cases to predictor ratio), three is much better than eight.

The eigen values (Table 5.9) are slightly smaller, suggesting less separation of the classes and the contribution made by the second function has declined. However, both functions retain some significant discriminatory power.

Table 5.9. *Summary of discriminant functions for golden eagle data using forward selection*

Function	Eigen value (λ)	Percentage of variance	Wilk's lambda	Chi-square	df	p	Canonical correlation
1	3.816	73.3	0.087	87.998	6	0.000	0.890
2	1.393	26.7	0.418	31.409	2	0.000	0.763

Table 5.10. *Standardised canonical discriminant function coefficients (only for selected predictors) and structure coefficients (correlations between discriminating variables and standardised canonical discriminant functions) for both discriminant functions. The largest absolute correlation between each predictor and any discriminant function is marked with an asterisk*

Predictor	Standardised canonical discriminant function coefficients		Structure coefficients	
	1	2	1	2
POST			-0.072^*	-0.037
PRE			0.046	0.088^*
BOG			-0.481^*	-0.269
CALL			-0.250	0.290^*
WET	0.084	-0.199	0.674^*	-0.577
STEEP	0.062	-0.159	0.339	-0.717^*
LT200	0.095	0.794	0.236	0.972^*
L4_600			0.049	-0.568^*

Although only three predictors have weights in the discriminant function all of the potential predictors have structure coefficients (Table 5.10). This is because the structure coefficients are simple correlation coefficients between the discriminant scores and the potential predictor values. Hence they can still be used to interpret differences between the regions.

Using the structure matrix for an interpretation of the differences between regions it appears that large positive scores on function one are mainly associated with large areas of wet heath and small areas of bog (negative correlation) while large positive scores on function two are mainly associated with large areas of land below 200 m and small areas of steep land, land between 400 and 600 m and wet heath. These are effectively the same axes that were obtained using all eight predictors. Since the axes are similar it is

Table 5.11. *Classification statistics for golden eagle range predictions using stepwise selection of predictors*

		Predicted class		
Classifier	Actual class	1	2	3
Re-substituted	1	7	0	0
	2	0	14	2
	3	0	0	17
Percentage cases correctly classified			95.0%	
Cross-validated	1	6	0	1
	2	0	14	2
	3	0	0	17
Percentage cases correctly classified			95.0%	

perhaps not too surprising that the separation is similar to the previous analysis (not shown here).

However, one may be surprised that the cross-validated classification accuracy is better using fewer predictors (Table 5.11). This is not as surprising as it sounds. Watanabe's (1985) 'ugly duckling' theorem states that adding sufficient irrelevant predictors can make cases from different classes more similar and hence degrade performance.

Although this stepwise analysis has produced some promising results, it can be criticised because it involved the rather unthinking application of a stepwise selection procedure. In the next example the predictors are selected via a more defensible process.

We are allowed to use some judgement in the selection of predictors. Indeed we should be encouraged to do so since it means that we are thinking more deeply about the problem. Huberty (1994) suggested three variable screening techniques that could be used with a discriminant analysis:

- Logical screening uses theoretical, reliability and practical grounds to screen variables.
- Statistical screening uses statistical tests to identify variables whose values differ significantly between groups. Huberty suggests applying a relaxed criterion, in that only predictors that are most likely to be 'noise' (e.g. $F < 1.0$ or $t < 1.0$) are rejected. In addition, the inter-predictor correlations should be examined to find those that are 'highly correlated'. Redundant predictors should be removed.

- Dimension reduction uses a method such as PCA (Section 2.5.2) to reduce the predictor dimensionality. This has the additional advantage of removing any predictor collinearity.

This example analysis concentrates on statistical screening and applies rather stricter criteria than Huberty suggests. This is because of the need to drastically prune the number of variables. The first step is to carry out a single-factor analysis of variance to find out which variables discriminate between the regions. The F statistics are used to rank the potential predictors. Two potential predictors, POST and CAL, have p values >0.05, and, if a Bonferroni correction for multiple testing is applied, the p value for PRE becomes insignificant. Consequently, these three are excluded. The rank order of retained predictors, based on F statistics is: WET ($F = 40.7$); LT200 ($F = 28.3$); STEEP ($F = 21.4$); BOG ($F = 18.4$); and L4_600 ($F = 8.1$).

The next stage is to examine the correlations between these five predictors. Not surprisingly, LT200 and L4_600 are highly correlated ($r = -0.700$). Since LT200 has the larger F statistic L4_600 is excluded. Similarly WET and STEEP are highly correlated ($r = 0.690$). For similar reasons STEEP is excluded. This leaves three predictors: WET, LT200 and BOG. BOG is reasonably correlated with the other two (-0.543 with WET and -0.314 with LT200), while WET and LT200 have an insignificant correlation ($r = -0.203$, $p = 0.209$). Therefore, BOG is excluded, leaving only WET and LT200. The desired two predictors (to fulfil the minimum cases:predictors ratio) are now used in a discriminant analysis. Note that these two predictors were the most important in the previous two analyses. As in the previous analyses two discriminant functions can be extracted (Table 5.12).

The first eigen value has decreased but the second is very similar to the previous analysis. However, both functions still retain some significant discriminatory power. The structure matrix (Table 5.13) suggests that the first function is mainly associated with wet heath (WET). Cases with a high positive score have more wet heath. The second function comprises both WET and LT200.

Table 5.12. *Summary of discriminant functions for golden eagle data using predictor screening*

Function	Eigen value (λ)	Percentage of variance	Wilk's lambda	Chi-square	df	p	Canonical correlation
1	2.930	68.3	0.108	81.286	4	0.000	0.863
2	1.359	31.7	0.424	31.327	1	0.000	0.759

Table 5.13. *Standardised canonical discriminant function coefficients (only for selected predictors) and structure coefficients (correlations between discriminating variables and standardised canonical discriminant functions) for both discriminant functions*

Predictor	Standardised canonical discriminant function coefficients		Structure coefficients	
	1	2	1	2
WET	1.033	−0.359	0.731	−0.682
LT200	0.746	0.800	0.328	0.945

Table 5.14. *Classification statistics for golden eagle range predictions using predictor screening*

Classifier	Actual class	Predicted class		
		1	2	3
Re-substituted	1	7	0	0
	2	1	12	3
	3	0	0	17
Percentage cases correctly classified			90.0%	
	1	7	0	0
Cross-validated	2	1	12	3
	3	0	0	17
Percentage cases correctly classified			90.0%	

Larger positive scores are associated with land that has less wet heath and more land below 200 m. As in the other analyses, function one separates regions 1 and 2, while function two separates region 3 from the rest.

This analysis, based on only two predictors, produces a better cross-validated discrimination (Table 5.14) than the first one using all eight. It is only marginally worse than the stepwise analysis with three predictors. Overall, this final analysis is more robust and involved a significant amount of preliminary exploratory analyses. This reinforces the point that there is usually little lost, and much to be gained, by spending time investigating the data before embarking on a final analysis.

5.3.3   *Modified algorithms*

Since the technique was developed by Fisher a variety of extensions to the basic algorithm have appeared. For example, flexible, mixture, penalised and quadratic discriminant analyses are all based on similar principles and all four are available as functions within the R analysis environment. Flexible discriminant analysis (Hastie *et al.*, 1994) is a generalisation that uses a non-parametric regression that creates non-linear decision boundaries. Mixture discriminant analysis (Hastie and Tibshirani, 1996) creates a classifier by fitting a Gaussian mixture model to each class. The reason for using a mixture model is that heterogeneous classes are poorly represented by the single 'prototypes' that characterise linear discriminant analysis; the mixture model allows multiple prototypes. A penalised discriminant analysis (Hastie *et al.*, 1995) attempts to overcome the collinearity problems created when many predictors are correlated by using a penalised regression. In a linear discriminant analysis the boundaries between the classes are flat. Quadratic discriminant analysis allows them to become curved quadratic surfaces. In a quadratic discriminant analysis there is no assumption that the covariance matrices are equal. While this can be an advantage it comes at a cost of an increase in the number of parameters, possibly leading to a greater chance of over-fitting the training data. Because of these risks, and the relatively robust nature of linear discriminant analysis (Gilbert, 1969), quadratic discrimination is only recommended when differences between the class covariance matrices are large (Marks and Dunn, 1974).

5.4   Logistic regression

5.4.1   Introduction

In a classification problem, where the dependent variable has only two possible values (e.g. zero and one) methods such as multiple regression become invalid because predicted values of *y* would not be constrained to lie between zero and one. Although discriminant analysis can be used in such circumstances it will only produce optimal solutions if its assumptions are supported by the data, which could be tested using an EDA. An alternative approach is logistic regression.

In logistic regression the dependent variable is the probability that an event will occur, and hence *y* is constrained between zero and one. It has the additional advantage that the predictors can be binary, a mixture of categorical and continuous or just continuous. Although categorical predictors can be used they are recoded as a series of dummy binary predictors. The number of dummy variables is always one less than the number of categories, otherwise there would be serious collinearity problems. This is the reason why a binary categorical variable such as gender is coded by a single 0/1 variable rather than separate 0/1 male and female variables. However, lack of independence (collinearity) between continuous predictors can still lead to biased estimates and inflated standard errors for the coefficients.

The logistic model, which is a GLM, is written as

$$P(\text{event}) = 1/(1 - e^{-z})$$

where z is $b_0 + b_1x_1 + b_2x_2 + \dots b_px_p$ and $P(\text{event})$ is the probability that a case belongs to a particular class, which is assumed to be the class with the value one. In this format, the relationship between $P(\text{event})$ and its predictors is non-linear. However, the logistic equation can be rearranged into a linear form by using a link function to convert the probability into a log odds or logit, where $\text{logit}[P(\text{event})] = \log[P(\text{event})/P(\text{no event})]$. There is a non-linear relationship between p and its logit. In the mid range of $P(\text{event})$ the relationship is linear, but as $P(\text{event})$ approaches the zero or one extremes the relationship becomes non-linear with increasingly larger changes in logit for the same change in p (Figure 5.6). Note that this transformation can also be written in a linear format: $\text{logit}(P(\text{event})) = \log P(\text{event}) - \log P(\text{no event})$.

The rearranged equation produces a linear relationship between the class and the predictors similar to that in multiple regression, $\text{logit}P(\text{event}) = b_0 + b_1x_1 + b_2x_2 + \dots b_px_p$. However, in this form each one-unit change in a predictor is associated with a change in log odds rather than the response directly. Many biologists find it difficult to interpret the coefficients from a logistic regression. This is not too surprising given that they relate to changes in $\text{logit}(p)$, rather than p itself. Because the logit transformation is non-linear the change in p, brought about by a one-unit change in the value of predictor, changes with the value

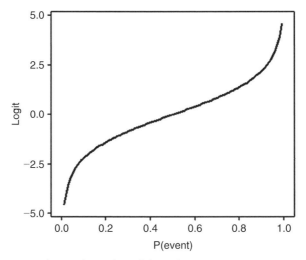

Figure 5.6 Logit transformation of $P(\text{event})$.

of the predictor. Consequently, it is worth examining the interpretation of log odds since they are so important to the method and yet simultaneously meaningless to many biologists!

Suppose that a logistic regression predicts presence (1) or absence (0) of some outcome using a set of three binary predictors (A, B and C), for example gender, smoking and colour blindness, where one indicates presence and zero absence of that predictor. The following equation was obtained: log odds $= -2.7 + 2.5\,A - 3.7\,B + 1.8\,C$. The coefficient of 2.5 for predictor A is the estimated change in the logarithm of $P(\text{presence})/P(\text{absence})$, when B and C are held constant.

If A, B and C are present (i.e. have the value 1) the log odds are: log odds $= -2.7 + 2.5 - 3.7 + 1.8 = -2.1$, giving odds of 0.1225 ($e^{-2.1}$). The 'risk' (probability of event 1) is defined as the odds ratio (odds/(1 + odds)). Odds ratios less than one correspond to decreases in the odds as the predictor increases in value while odds ratios greater than one correspond to increases in the odds. If the odds ratio is approximately one, changes in the predictor do not alter the probability of the event. Note that a coefficient of zero is the same as an odds ratio of one (because e^{-0} is 1.0), both imply the predictor has no effect of the response. In this example the odds, when all predictors have a value of one, are equal to 0.1225/1.1225 or 0.1091 (10.91%). If A, B and C are absent, and have the value zero, then the log odds equal the constant. In this example the constant is -2.7 giving log odds of -2.7 and odds of 0.067 ($e^{-2.7}$). This means that 'risk' of event 1 is 0.067/1.067 or 0.063 (6.3%). Therefore, absence of the three predictors almost halves the chance of the event. However, if predictors A and C are present, while B is absent, the log odds are $-2.7 + 2.5 + 1.8 = 1.6$, giving odds of 4.953 ($e^{1.6}$) and a risk of 4.953/5.953 = 0.832 or 83.2%. It appears that the absence of predictor B vastly increases the probability of event 1.

Similar calculations can be performed for continuous predictors. The relevant predictor values are 'plugged' into the equation and multiplied by their weights to give the log odds. This means that each one-unit increase in a predictor (e.g. a change from 78 kg to 79 kg) will change the log odds by the value of the coefficient. It is for this reason that statistical software often report exp(b) values (e^{b}) in addition to the coefficient.

The logistic equation can be used to estimate the probability of an event for each case. These probabilities can then be used to assign each case to a class by the application of some threshold to its probability. This means that the continuously valued probabilities are discretised into a binary class variable. The default threshold is 0.5, so cases will be assigned to the 'event' class if their probability of being in that class is estimated to be >0.5. While this may seem reasonable there are problems, some of which relate to the tendency of techniques, such as logistic regression, to assign preferentially cases to the largest class. This is discussed in much more detail in Chapter 7. Nonetheless, it is usual to present a summary table, similar to that used with discriminant analysis, of class allocations against actual class.

Dettling and Bühlmann (2004) describe a penalised extension to normal logistic regression that they apply to microarray data, specifically to deal with the excess of predictors that is common in such classification problems. Their method combines variable selection and extraction with class allocation.

It is undoubtedly true that one has to think more carefully about what the results from a logistic mean, but that is no bad thing. Hosmer and Lemeshow (1994) is the standard text on logistic regression and should be consulted if one intends using this method in research.

5.4.2   Example analyses
Artificial data

This analysis uses the second data set (B) from Section 5.3.2 (see Appendix E) and will, therefore, enable a direct comparison with the discriminant analyses of the same data. The analysis was completed using SPSS^{TM} version 12.0. No stepwise predictor selection methods were used and all of the predictors are continuous variables. Recall that, individually, all four predictors are good predictors of the class but that b4 is highly correlated with b3, while all other between-predictor correlations are insignificant.

The results begin with a summary of the final model which includes log-likelihood (-2 LL), a measure of the goodness of fit, and pseudo-R^2 statistics which measure the variability in the dependent variable (the class) that is explained by the predictors. Because the usual least squares R^2 statistic cannot be calculated a range of pseudo-R^2 statistics have been designed to provide similar information. SPSS reports two, the first being the Cox and Snell statistic (1989, pp. 208−9) which tends not to have the desired 0−1 range because its maximum is usually less than one. Nagelkerke's R^2 (1991) is derived from the previous one, but with a guarantee of a 0−1 range. Consequently it tends to have larger values. Values close to zero are associated with models that do not provide much information about the probability of class memberships. In this analysis they are quite large (0.439 and 0.585) suggesting that over half of the variation in classes can be explained by the current predictors.

The log-likelihood (LL) is a measure of the variation in the response variable that is unexplained by the model. LLs are the logarithms of probabilities and, since probabilities are never greater than one, the logarithm will be negative. If the LL is multiplied by -2 (-2LL) the resulting measure, which is often called the deviance, approximates to a chi-square statistic and can be used to test hypotheses. At the start of the logistic modelling process the simplest model, the null model, has one term, the intercept or constant. Large values for the deviance measure indicate a poor fit because there is a large amount of unexplained variation. As the model is developed, i.e. predictors are added, it is expected that deviance will decline. At the start of this model the deviance was 207.9, suggesting a very poor fit. The final model has a deviance of 121.3. This means that the change in the deviance has been $207.9 - 121.3 = 86.6$. SPSS calls this the model chi-square and it is used to test a hypothesis that the predictors have improved the model by reducing the amount of unexplained variation. Since $p \ll 0.05$ there is strong evidence that the model, which includes the four predictors, has significantly reduced the unexplained variation.

The Hosmer−Lemeshow statistic is often used to estimate the goodness-of-fit of the model. The number of cases in ten groups, ordered by their probabilities (observed values), are compared with the numbers in each group predicted by the logistic regression model (predicted values). Since this is a comparison of observed and expected frequencies, the test statistic is a chi-square statistic with eight degrees of freedom. If the differences are not significant it indicates that the model prediction does not differ significantly from the observed. This is the desired outcome. In this analysis the value of chi-square is 2.495, giving a p value of >0.9, which provides further strong evidence for a good fit.

The structure of a model is determined by the coefficients and their significance (Table 5.15). The Wald statistic also has an approximate chi-square distribution and is used to determine if the coefficients are significantly different from zero. In a least squares regression the significance of the coefficients is usually tested with a t-statistic, which is the coefficient divided by its standard error. In Table 5.20 a similar test is used to derive a z-value for the coefficients. Wald's statistic is obtained by a similar calculation but, because it is a chi-squared measure the ratio is squared. For example, the Wald statistic for b1 is 19.351,

Table 5.15. *Regression coefficients. The Wald statistic has one degree of freedom. The upper and lower confidence limits refer to Exp(B)*

Predictor	b	s.e.	Wald	P	Exp(B)	95% LCL	95% UCL
b1	0.511	0.116	19.351	0.000	1.667	1.328	2.094
b2	0.355	0.080	19.675	0.000	1.427	1.219	1.669
b3	0.349	0.084	17.191	0.000	1.418	1.202	1.672
b4	−0.062	0.043	2.108	0.147	0.940	0.864	1.022
Constant	−17.49	2.856	37.483	0.000	0.000		

which is $(0.51123/0.11622)^2$. Unfortunately, the Wald statistic can be unreliable because larger coefficients tend to have inflated standard errors, meaning that the chi-square statistic is reduced leading to a larger p value (Hauck and Donner, 1977). The significance of the coefficients can also be judged from the confidence limits for exp(b). Recall that a predictor which has no effect on the response will have odds (exp(b)) of 1.0. Therefore, if the confidence limits include one, see b4 in Table 5.15, there is no evidence for a relationship between the predictor and the event. In this example it should be remembered that the lack of significance for b4 is related to its correlation with b3. Indeed, when used as a single predictor its coefficient is significantly different from zero and the confidence limits for exp(b) do not include 1.

The classification results (Table 5.16) are almost identical to the discriminant analysis predictions (Table 5.3). Indeed there is little difference between the two analyses, with the three significant predictors having similar proportional values for their coefficients.

Mixed data type analysis

The previous data set could have been analysed using discriminant analysis because all of the predictors were continuous. However, it becomes more difficult to use discriminant analysis when predictors are categorical. The second logistic regression analysis uses data collected from 87 people (Appendix G). The response variable is whether or not a person smokes (66 non-smokers and 21 smokers) and the five predictors consist of two categorical (gender and ABO blood type) and three continuous (age (years); body mass index, bmi (kg m^{-2}); white blood cell count, wbc ($\times 10^9 1^{-1}$)) predictors. Because gender has two values it is coded as a single binary predictor (0 = male, 1 = female). Blood group has four categories that must be coded as three dummy predictors. The coding is arbitrary and is shown in Table 5.17. Blood group AB has an implicit coding of zero for each of the three dummy blood group predictors.

Table 5.16. *Classification table (using a 0.5 threshold)*

Actual class	Predicted class		Percentage correct
	1	2	
1	61	14	81.3
2	14	61	81.3
Overall percentage			81.3

Table 5.17. *ABO blood group categorical codings into three binary predictors*

ABO type	Frequency	Parameter coding		
		(1)	(2)	(3)
O	21	1	0	0
A	24	0	1	0
B	22	0	0	1
AB	20	0	0	0

Table 5.18. *Regression coefficients. The Wald statistic has one degree of freedom. The upper and lower confidence limits refer to Exp(B)*

Predictor	b	s.e.	Wald	p	Exp(B)	95% LCL	95% UCL
bmi	−0.214	0.096	4.942	0.026	0.807	0.669	0.975
wbc	0.632	0.214	8.705	0.003	1.882	0.958	0.669
age	0.031	0.038	0.682	0.409	1.032	1.236	2.864
sex(1)	−0.188	0.615	0.094	0.760	0.829	0.248	2.764
abo			3.685	0.298			
abo(1)	−1.290	0.885	2.124	0.145	0.275	0.049	1.560
abo(2)	−0.430	0.762	0.319	0.572	0.651	0.146	2.895
abo(3)	−1.335	0.814	2.688	0.101	0.263	0.053	1.298
Constant	−0.034	2.775	0.000	0.990	0.967		

The null model has only the intercept, whose initial value is $\log_e(P(\text{smoke})/P(\text{non-smoke}))$. The deviance for the null model is 96.164, which reduces to 75.8 when all of the predictors are added. The reduction in the deviance (20.371) is significant ($p = 0.005$) suggesting that the predictors significantly reduce the unexplained variation. This is further supported by the pseudo-R^2 values, although values around 0.3 indicate that a large amount of variation remains unexplained by these predictors.

As may be expected, both age and blood group are not good predictors of smoking habits (Table 5.18). It is less obvious, a priori, if gender should be a predictor. In these data gender does not predict smoking. The only two significant predictors are bmi and wbc. The probability of smoking appears to decline as bmi increases, suggesting that given two people of the same height, but different weights, the lighter person is more likely to smoke. The coefficient for wbc is positive, suggesting that the probability that a person smokes is greater if their white blood cell count is larger. Indeed there is a well-known

Table 5.19. *Classification table (using a 0.5 threshold) for predicting the smoking habitats of people from a sample of 87 cases*

Actual class	Predicted class		Percentage correct
	N	Y	
N	62	4	93.9
Y	12	9	42.9
Overall percentage			81.6

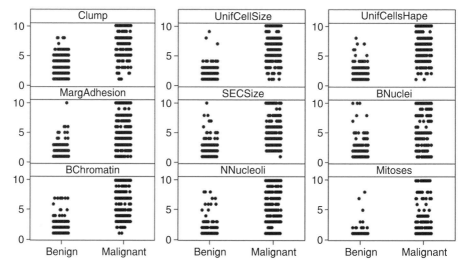

Figure 5.7 Individual value plots for the nine predictors (clump thickness, Clump; uniformity of cell size, UnifCellSize; uniformity of cell shape, UnifCellShape; marginal adhesion, MargAdhesion; single epithelial cell size, SECSize; bare nuclei, BNuclei; bland chromatin, BChromatin; nucleoli, NNucleoli; and Mitoses).

relationship for white blood cell counts to be higher in smokers (e.g. Kannel *et al.*, 1992).

The classification results (Table 5.19) suggest that, despite the significance of the predictors, the model tends to predict smokers incorrectly, a problem which is at least partly related to the large difference in the proportions of smokers and non-smokers. If the class allocation threshold is adjusted (from 0.50 to 0.28) to match the class proportions in the sample data the overall accuracy declines to 73.6% but the number of smokers correctly predicted rises from 9/21 to 14/21. The decline in overall accuracy is a consequence of more false identifications of non-smokers as smokers. Possible solutions to the problems created by unequal class proportions are covered in more detail in Chapter 7.

5.4.3   Cancer data set

Background

The final analysis uses the same data set as that used in Section 3.9.3. It is also used as an example in the next section which deals with generalised additive models. There are nine continuous potential predictor variables plus one class variable (benign, malignant). The predictors are: clump thickness; uniformity of cell size; uniformity of cell shape; marginal adhesion; single epithelial cell size; bare nuclei; bland chromatin; nucleoli; and mitoses. Figure 5.7 shows how the classes are separated by the predictors. By way of comparison with the previous analysis this one used the *glm* function within R.

Analysis

The deviance of the null model is 884.3, which reduces to 102.9 for the full model. This reduction is highly significant. The model coefficients and their significance levels (Table 5.20) suggest that four of the predictors have coefficients that differ significantly from zero: bland chromatin; bare nuclei; clump thickness; and marginal adhesion.

Figure 5.8 illustrates a graphical way of visualising the relationships between the cancer class and the predictors. These effect plots show, with confidence limits, the estimated relationship between the probability of belonging to the malignant class and the value of a potential predictor. Note that some of the insignificant predictors, for example mitoses, have quite large coefficients but they are combined with wide confidence limits.

Table 5.20. *Model coefficients and 95% confidence limits*

Predictor	Coefficient (b)	s.e.	LCL	UCL	z value	$Pr(>|z|)$	Exp(b)
(Intercept)	−10.1039	1.17488	−12.7584	−8.08641	−8.600	<0.0001	
Bland chromatin	0.4472	0.17138	0.1232	0.79993	2.609	0.0091	1.564
Bare nuclei	0.3830	0.09384	0.2069	0.57875	4.082	<0.0001	1.467
Clump thickness	0.5350	0.14202	0.2742	0.83781	3.767	0.0002	1.707
Marginal adhesion	0.3306	0.12345	0.0930	0.58702	2.678	0.0074	1.392
Mitoses	0.5348	0.32877	−0.0042	1.10624	1.627	0.1038	1.707
Nucleoli	0.2130	0.11287	−0.0018	0.44563	1.887	0.0591	1.237
Single epithelial cell size	0.0966	0.15659	−0.2169	0.40490	0.617	0.5372	1.101
Uniformity of cell shape	0.3227	0.23060	−0.1483	0.76840	1.399	0.1617	1.381
Uniformity of cell size	−0.0063	0.20908	−0.3948	0.43803	−0.030	0.9760	0.994

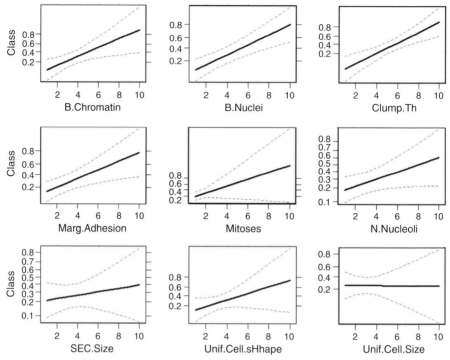

Figure 5.8 Effect plots for the cancer data, showing 95% confidence limits for the best fit lines (Clump.Th, clump thickness; uniformity of cell size, Unif.Cell.Size; uniformity of cell shape, Unif.Cell.Shape; marginal adhesion, Marg.Adhesion; single epithelial cell size, SEC.Size; bare nuclei, B.Nuclei; bland chromatin, B.Chromatin; N.Nucleoli, nucleoli; and mitoses).

Table 5.21. *Classification table (using a 0.5 threshold) for predicting the type of cancer from a large sample of cases*

Actual class	Predicted class		Percentage correct
	Benign	Malignant	
Benign	434	11	97.5
Malignant	10	228	95.8
Overall percentage			96.9

The logistic regression appears to be quite accurate, correctly predicting the class of most cases (Table 5.21). It would be worth examining the small number of misclassified cases to determine, if possible, what other characters have kept them out of their predicted class.

Residuals and influence statistics

In any regression analysis, including a logistic regression, it is important to check that there are no problems created by one or more of the cases that may invalidate the model. For example, if a case is substantially different from the rest it could have a large effect on the structure of the regression model. It is important to be aware of this so that it can be investigated further. In the simplest situation it could be that a value has been entered incorrectly, which, when corrected, removes its influence. Usually such investigations depend on calculating various diagnostic statistics such as residuals and influence statistics. Hosmer and Lemeshow (1989) suggest that these diagnostic statistics should be interpreted jointly to understand any potential problems with the model. The aim is to identify cases that are either outliers or have a large leverage. An outlier is an observation with a response value that is unusual, given the values for its predictor variables. This will result in it having a large residual, the difference between its actual and predicted value. Conversely a case could have an unusually small or large value for one of the predictors, which may cause it to have a disproportionate effect on the regression coefficient estimates. The size of this effect is measured as the leverage of a case, a measure of how far its value for a predictor deviates from the predictor's mean. The combination of leverage and outlying values can produce cases that have a large influence. These cases can be recognised because their removal results in large changes to the values of the regression coefficients. However, it also important to recognise that a case with a large leverage need not have a large residual. Hence the need to consider both together.

There are a surprisingly large number of diagnostic statistics, including many types of residual. For example, unstandardised residuals are the simple differences between the observed and predicted values of the response while standardised residuals (also known as Pearson or chi residuals) are the standardised residuals divided by an estimate of their standard deviation (actual value minus its predicted probability, divided by the binomial standard deviation of the predicted probability). Using the standard deviation as a devisor changes their probability distribution so that they have a standard deviation of one. There are other residuals such as the logit residual which measures the difference between actual and predicted values on the logit scale and the studentised residual which is the change in the model deviance if a case is excluded.

Because the standardised and studentised residuals, at least for large samples, should approximate to a normal distribution with a mean of zero and a standard deviation of one, no more than 5% of the residuals should exceed $|1.96|$ or approximately two. Similarly, less than 1% of the residuals should exceed $|3.0|$.

There are three main statistics that assess the influence that an individual case has on the model. The first is the leverage (h) of a case, which varies from zero (no influence) to one (completely determines the model). The second statistic, Cook's distance (D), also measures the influence of an observation by estimating how much all the other residuals would change if the case was removed. Its value is a function of the case's leverage and of the magnitude of its standardised residual. Normally, $D > 1.0$ identifies cases that might be influential. Dfbeta, or dbeta, is Cook's distance, standardised and it measures the change in the logit coefficients when a case is removed. As with D, an arbitrary threshold criterion for cases with poor fit is dfbeta > 1.0.

In this analysis the histogram of standardised residuals (Figure 5.9) does not suggest too many problems. Six cases (Table 5.22) have large standardised residuals, but this is within the expected number of large residuals.

A plot of Cook's D highlights several cases with large values, but only two cases (191 and 245) have values greater than one (Figure 5.10). Both of these cases are also highlighted in Table 5.22 as having large standardised residuals. These cases have large values for all predictors, suggesting that their true classification should be malignant and not benign. In practice, it would be worth spending time investigating these cases and verifying, at a minimum, that the predictor and class details were correct.

5.5   Discriminant analysis or logistic regression?

There have been many studies comparing logistic regression and discriminant analysis. Unfortunately the results of the comparisons are inconclusive.

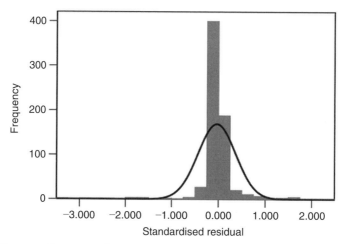

Figure 5.9 Frequency distribution of standardised residuals with an overlaid normal distribution.

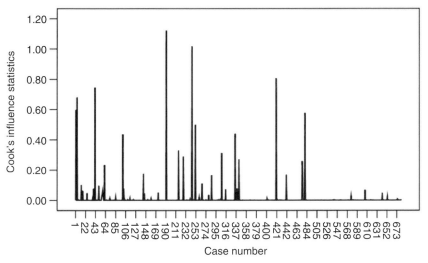

Figure 5.10 Cook's *D* statistic plotted against case number.

Table 5.22. *Cases with a standardised residual greater than two*

Case	Class	Predicted value	Predicted class	Residual	Standardised residual
2	Benign	0.909	Malignant	−0.909	−2.25
100	Malignant	0.137	Benign	0.863	2.06
191	Benign	0.998	Malignant	−0.998	−3.49
217	Malignant	0.047	Benign	0.953	2.49
245	Benign	0.979	Malignant	−0.979	−2.81
420	Benign	0.963	Malignant	−0.963	−2.60

The only universal criterion for selecting logistic regression over discriminant analysis relates to the data type limitations of discriminant analysis. Because both methods construct linear boundaries between the classes they have a similar functional form (a sum of weighted predictors). However, they differ in their assumptions about probability distributions and the methods used to estimate the predictor weights. Logistic regression does not make the same restrictive assumptions about predictor probability distributions, while discriminant analysis has a formal assumption of normally distributed predictors. Logistic regression uses a maximum likelihood method while discriminant analysis uses a least squares technique. One consequence of the different assumptions is that discriminant analysis should outperform logistic regression, when its assumptions are valid, while, in other circumstances, logistic regression should be the better option. However, empirical tests of the assumptions do not always support these conclusions. As long as the predictors are not categorical there appears to be little difference between the performance of the two methods when sample sizes are reasonable (> 50). If there are outliers it is likely that logistic regression will be better because the outliers could distort the variance–covariance matrix used in the estimation of predictor weights by discriminant analysis.

5.6   Generalised additive models

5.6.1   *Introduction*

Generalized additive models (GAMs) are also extensions of the general linear model but, unlike generalised linear models, they are semi-parametric rather than fully parametric. This is because the link function is a non-parametric 'smoothed' function and the form of the smoothing function is determined by the data rather than some pre-defined theoretical relationship. This is why a GAM is known as a data-driven, rather than a model-driven, algorithm. Despite this flexibility, they are semi-parametric rather than non-parametric, because the probability distribution of the response variable (the class in a classifier) must still be specified. In a GAM the simple coefficients (weights) are replaced by non-parametric relationships that are typically modelled using smoothing functions (Section 5.6.2). This produces models in which $g(L) = \Sigma s_i(x_i)$, where the $s_i(x_i)$ terms are the smoothed functions. The GAM is therefore a more general form of the generalised linear model. Although they have some advantages over simple polynomial regressions, they are more complicated to fit, and require a greater user judgement in their design. Also, although they may produce better predictions, they may be difficult to interpret.

The main advantage of GAMs is that they can deal with highly non-linear and non-monotonic relationships between the class and the predictors. General linear and linearised models can sometimes be improved, to deal with the non-linearity, by applying transformations, or including polynomial terms of the predictors. These transformations are generally not needed in a GAM because the smoothing function effectively carries out the transformation automatically. In this respect the smoothing functions are similar to the hidden layer in an artificial neural network (Chapter 6).

5.6.2   *Loess and spline smoothing functions*

Smoothing functions are central to the GAM approach because they produce a line, which need not be straight or even monotonic, to describe the general relationship between a pair of variables. Two of the most common methods, loess and the related lowess, derive their names from the term 'LOcally

WEighted Scatter plot Smooth'. They are locally weighted linear regression analyses that find arbitrarily complex (non-parametric) relationships between two variables. In effect they 'smooth' the relationship. They differ from normal regression methods because they do not look for a global relationship but build up a series of neighbourhoods defined by a span or neighbourhood size. Loess and lowess differ in the order of the local regression with loess using a quadratic, or second degree, polynomial and lowess a linear polynomial.

The fit between the two variables, y and x, at point x is estimated using points within a span or neighbourhood of s. These points are weighted by their distance from x. Normally, the span is specified as a percentage of the number of data points. For example, a span of 0.25 uses a quarter of the data points. Typically case weights become smaller as data points become more distant from x. The central data point within the span, x, has the largest weight and the most influence on the fit, while cases outside the span have zero weight and hence no effect on the local fit. The size of the span affects the complexity of the smoothed relationship, with larger spans giving smoother fits (see Figure 5.11). If the span is too small the 'smoothing' will model the random error in the data, while spans that are too large may miss important local trends. These are the same over-fitting problems that may arise in artificial

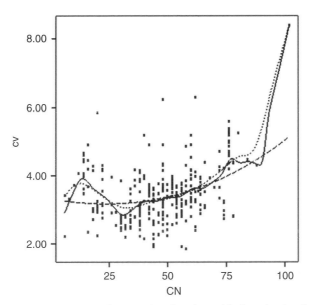

Figure 5.11 Example use of a smoother function with three levels of smoothing. Data are from Gregory (2005) and relate to mammalian genome size. CV, haploid C-value (in pg); CN, diploid chromosome number (2n).

neural networks and decision trees (Chapter 6). Useful values of the smoothing parameter typically lie in the range 0.25 to 0.75.

There are other smoothing algorithms such the B-spline smoother (Hastie, 1992) used as the default by the *gam* function in R. The fit of the line to the data points is measured as the sum of square deviations between actual and fitted values of the response, where the fitted values are obtained from local curve-fitting routines. For example, the spline smoother fits a series of piecewise polynomials. However, unless some constraint is applied the resulting curve could be too 'wiggly'. A curve that is too complex is almost certainly capturing noise from the data rather than the overall trend. Conversely, a line that is too simple, for example a straight line, would fail to capture any non-linearity in the relationship. Therefore, a compromise is required that balances the minimisation of the squared deviations with the need to avoid an over-complex line. This is achieved by incorporating a penalty term. In the R implementation the degree of smoothness is controlled by specifying the effective degrees of freedom, which is then used to adjust the penalty term. If four degrees of freedom are specified this is equivalent to a third-degree polynomial, while one degree of freedom would fit the smoother as a simple straight line. The rationale behind choosing the appropriate degrees of freedom for smoothers is discussed in detail by Hastie and Tibshirani (1990). It is important that an appropriate degree of smoothing is selected because over-complex smoothers will generate false optimism about the classifier's future performance. This is discussed further in Chapter 7.

5.6.3   *Example analysis*

These analyses were carried out using the *gam* function from R. Because the degree of smoothing is one of the most important parameters in the GAM analysis three analyses are described. The first two use the default B-spline smoother with four and seven degrees of freedom. A relatively large value of seven was chosen because it is likely to produce a function that over-fits the data and begins to model noise in the relationships between the cancer class and the predictors. The third uses a loess smoother with a span of 0.75. Figure 5.12 illustrates how an adjustment to the degree of smoothing can alter the interpretation of the model. As the fitted curve becomes more complex the predictor changes from having an insignificant to a significant effect.

The second model, with the more complex smoothed curves, has a much lower residual deviance than the other two models (Table 5.23). Each model has the same number of predictors but the degree of smoothing differs. As the smoothed curves become more complex they use up degrees of freedom, hence the least complex smoother has an additional 27 degrees of freedom. The loess smoothed model has the largest number of residual degrees of freedom. These differences

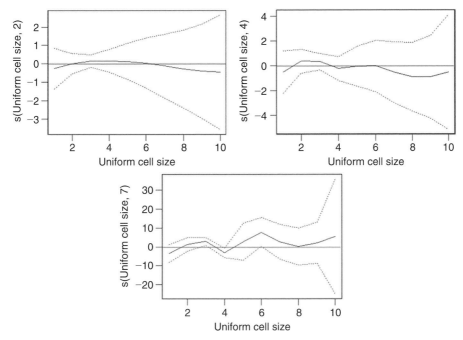

Figure 5.12 Partial effect plots for the uniform cell size predictor using two, four and seven as the smoothing parameter for the spline smoother. Note the different scales on the *y*-axes. Chi-square (and *p*) values for each function were 1.55 (0.21), 4.20 (0.24) and 12.84 (0.04).

Table 5.23. *Model deviance statistics for three GAM models with different smoothing factors. Also shown are the results from the previous logistic regression. The null deviance is 884.4, with 682 degrees of freedom, for all four models*

Model	Residual deviance (df)	AIC
B-spline smoother = 4	54.86 (646)	128.9
B-spline smoother = 7	4.5 (618.9)	132.5
Loess smoother (span = 0.75)	73.79 (657.9)	123.8
Logistic regression	102.9 (673)	122.9

become apparent if the AIC (Akaike's information criterion) is examined. The AIC is defined as $-2\log(L(\theta|\text{data})) + 2k$ (or $-2(\text{LL}) + 2k$), where $L(\theta|\text{data})$ is the likelihood of the parameters given the data and k is the number of parameters that are estimated during the model's development. In a simple model this could be the number of predictor coefficients plus the intercept. The log-likelihood is a measure of a model's fit. The AIC is useful because it penalises models for the addition of extra parameters which, in the case of GAM, will include the extra terms needed to provide the smoothed fit. The AIC is used to select, between models, the one which has a good fit but with the minimum number of parameters. It is often used in stepwise methods and information theoretic model comparison (ITMC) approaches. Because these analyses used the same data it is possible to rank them. However, it is important to understand that the AIC only provides information about the rank order of the tested models; it does not identify models that are the best of all possible (and untried) models. There is little to choose between the logistic regression and loess smoothed GAM. However, the two spline-smoothed GAMs seem to be considerably worse. Delta AICs (AIC − minimum AIC) are preferred to raw AIC values because they force the best, of the tested models, to have a Delta AIC of zero and thereby allow meaningful comparisons without the scaling issues that affect the AIC (Burnham and Anderson, 2004). It is also important not to compare the Delta AIC values to the raw AIC values because the raw values contain large scaling constants that are eliminated in the Delta AIC values (Burnham and Anderson, 2004). The Delta AIC values for these two models are 6.0 and 9.6, respectively. Burnham and Anderson (2002) suggest that Delta AIC values between three and seven indicate that the model has little support, and larger values reduce the support even further. Consequently, the best of these four models is the logistic one, although there is little difference from the loess smoothed GAM. Further information on the use of the AIC, and the related BIC (Bayesian information criterion), can be obtained from a Burnham and Anderson (2004) online conference paper.

Table 5.24. *Chi-square values for non-parametric effects from two GAM analyses using two smoothing levels (4 and 7)*

Predictor	B-spline smoother = 4 (df = 3)		B-spline smoother = 7 (df = 6)		Loess smoother (span = 0.75) df =	
	Chi-square	P(chi)	Chi-square	P(chi)	Chi-square	P(chi)
Clump thickness	4.80	0.19	8.87	0.18	8.88	0.18
Uniformity of cell size	4.20	0.24	12.84	0.06	12.39	0.06
Uniformity of cell shape	3.10	0.38	9.03	0.17	9.18	0.16
Marginal adhesion	9.16	0.03	24.96	0.00	25.40	0.00
Single epithelial cell size	10.70	0.01	20.99	0.00	20.41	0.00
Bare nuclei	5.21	0.16	17.31	0.01	17.17	0.01
Bland chromatin	3.75	0.29	8.66	0.19	8.93	0.18
Nucleoli	7.48	0.06	8.60	0.20	8.63	0.19
Mitoses	1.14	0.77	0.02	1.00	0.07	1.00

Table 5.24 gives the results, for each smoothing effect in the model, from a chi-square test that compares the deviance between the full model and the model without the variable. The results suggest that the effects of marginal adhesion and single epithelial cell size are significant in all three analyses, while the number of bare nuclei is also significant when the spline smoother is allowed to become more complex or the loess smoother is used. Marginal adhesion and bare nuclei were also significant predictors in the logistic regression model. The other two significant predictors from the logistic model, bland chromatin and clump thickness, were not close to being significant in any of the three GAM models.

The partial predictions for each predictor, from the third model with the loess smoother, are plotted in Figure 5.13. If a predictor is insignificant the confidence limits cover the line in which $y = 0$. The partial predictions also highlight the potentially non-linear nature of some of the relationships. This information

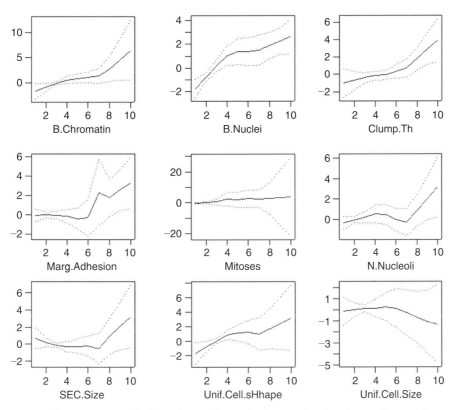

Figure 5.13 Partial effect plots, with standard errors, for the nine predictors using a loess smoother with a span of 0.75.

could be used to refine a generalised linear model by, for example, including quadratic terms for some of the predictors in a logistic regression. Bland chromatin and clump thickness, which are both significant in the logistic regression model, appear to have approximately linear relationships with the class, but the wider confidence intervals include zero and stop them from being significant.

The logistic regression model incorrectly predicted 21 cases. Two of the three GAM models performed slightly better with 12 (spline with a smoothing parameter of four) and 17 (loess smoother) incorrect. The other model correctly classified all cases. However, the errors do not relate to the same cases. For example, the first GAM model produced different predictions for eight cases compared with the logistic regression. There is little difference between these results and those using a discriminant analysis which incorrectly classifies 25 cases using re-substituted data and 26 cases from the cross-validated data. The 100% accuracy of the second GAM model should be treated with caution because of its large AIC and Delta AIC plus the factors explored in Chapter 7.

Although the GAM models are more accurate than the equivalent logistic regression model, the relationships are harder to interpret and it is more difficult to make predictions (although there is an option within the R *gam* function). For example, the significant, non-linear, non-monotonic relationship between the class and the amount of marginal adhesion shown in Figure 5.13 is difficult to explain.

5.7   Summary

Most of this chapter has focused on three statistical approaches that belong to the general class of linear models. Two of the methods, logistic regression and discriminant analysis, are 'old' methods, with the GAM approach being much more recent. There was little to choose between them with the cancer data, but this could just reflect the rather simple structure of these data. It is noted in Chapter 3 that even an unsupervised method performed well on these data. In the next chapter a range of methods, of more recent origin, is described. When comparing old and new methods it is important to be aware of the range of criteria on which they can be judged (see Section 7.9).

6

Other classification methods

6.1   Background

Despite their differences the classifiers in the previous chapter share a common ancestry – the general linear model. Consequently, they have similar relationships between the class and the predictors, albeit mediated via a link function that is determined by a defined class probability distribution. The estimated values of the predictor coefficients are found using maximum likelihood methods and tests are available to determine if they differ significantly from zero. In this chapter the methods share little in common with each other or the previous methods. Two methods are biologically inspired while a third has much in common with species identification keys. The other methods appear to work well but are less used in biology at the moment. The most important shared benefit, and potential problem, for the methods described in this chapter is that they are data-driven rather than model-driven. This can be an advantage in a knowledge-poor environment but it may come with the disadvantage that their structure is difficult to interpret. Many of these algorithms have features that reduce their susceptibility to noise and missing values, making them potentially valuable when dealing with 'real' data.

6.2   Decision trees

6.2.1   Background

Anyone who has used a species identification key should be familiar with the concept of a decision tree. Class labels are assigned to cases by following a path through a series of simple rules or questions, the answers to which determine the next direction through the pathway. The various decision tree algorithms create the rules from the information contained within the predictors. Superficially there is some similarity with a hierarchical, divisive, cluster analysis but there is an important and fundamental difference. Cluster analyses are unsupervised methods that take no account of pre-assigned class labels. A decision tree is a supervised learning algorithm which must be provided with a training set that contains cases with class labels.

The basic classification or decision tree algorithm is relatively simple. It begins with all of the cases in one group or node, known as the root node. All of the predictor variables are examined to find a decision, or split, that best separates out the classes. In a binary tree each split produces a left and a right node. Each of these nodes is then examined to determine if it should be split again. If it is to be split all of the predictors, including those used in earlier decisions, are examined again to find the best split. If the node is not split it becomes a terminal, or leaf, node and all of the cases in the node are labelled as belonging to the same class. Figure 6.1 illustrates this process using the *Iris* data described in Section 2.10.

The root node (0), which contains all of the training cases, is split using a petal length of 2.09 cm. Any flower with a smaller value goes into the left terminal node (1). This node is terminal because it contains only *I. setosa* individuals and there is no need to split it again. Individuals from the other two species are placed in the node to the right (2). This is split using a petal width criterion of 1.64 cm. The left node (3, flower width < 1.64) contains 48 *I. versicolor* and 4 *I. virginica* cases. The right node (4, flower width > 1.64) contains 2 *I. versicolor* and 46 *I. virginica* cases. Although neither of these nodes contains just one species, the algorithm stops so all cases in the left node are labelled as *I. versicolor* and all in the right node are labelled as *I. virginica*. This means that six out of 150 cases are incorrectly labelled. Once constructed, the decision tree can also be written as one or more rules. For example, the tree in Figure 6.1 can be described by the following rule:

```
If (petal length < 2.09 cm) then species = Iris setosa
Else
  If (petal width < 1.64 cm) then species = Iris versicolor
Else
  species = Iris virginica.
```

Because only two predictors are used in this tree it can be represented graphically with lines making the splits (Figure 6.2). Because the splits are usually univariate the decision boundaries in most decision trees are constrained to be axis-parallel. For example, the horizontal line in Figure 6.2 is the first split (petal length < 2.09). The univariate splits are an important difference from

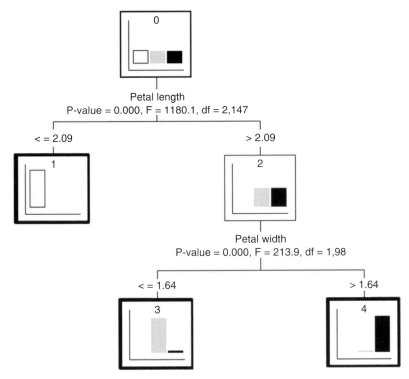

Figure 6.1 Decision tree for predicting the species of *Iris* from four floral characteristics. The tree was produced using SPSS™ AnswerTree Version 3.0. The bars represent the relative frequency of each species within a node (white bar; *I. setosa*; grey bar; *I. versicolor*; black bar; *I. virginica*).

the classifiers described in the previous chapter. Their decision boundaries, although flat, were not constrained to be axis-parallel. There are decision trees (see Section 6.2.4) that overcome this restriction by using multivariate decision rules. It is also important to realise that the lines which partition the predictor space are localised. For example, the second split in Figure 6.2 only applies to flowers with a petal length greater than 2.09 cm.

The simple outline described above avoids a lot of detail, much of which characterises the different 'flavours' of decision trees. It also explains why the method has the alternative name of recursive partitioning. At each decision point, or node, the data are partitioned. Each of these partitions is then partitioned independently of all other partitions, until some ending criterion is reached, in which case the node becomes a terminal, or leaf, node.

The two most important stages in the algorithm are identifying the best splits and determining when a node is terminal. In an ideal tree all terminal nodes

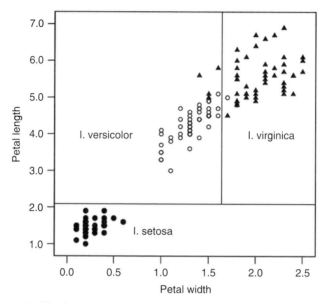

Figure 6.2 Simple decision tree presented as axis-parallel splits.

would be 'pure', meaning that all of the cases in a terminal node came from the same class. Two of the three terminal nodes in Figure 6.1 are impure, only node one is pure. It is generally possible, although not always desirable, to generate a tree in which most or all of the terminal nodes are pure. A tree such as that, which achieves 100% accuracy with the training data, is likely to have a complex structure which reflects the particular characteristics of the training data, rather than the general differences between the classes. For example, the *I. versicolor* node (3) can be split using another petal length criterion (< 5.24 cm) to produce two new terminal nodes: one pure node with 2 *I. virginica* cases and one impure node with 48 *I. versicolor* and 4 *I. virginica* cases. The need to retain some generality is the reason why accuracy must be balanced against complexity when deciding if impure nodes should be split further.

In certain circumstances decision trees have an advantage over more common supervised learning methods such as discriminant analysis. In particular, they do not have to conform to the same probability distribution restrictions. There is also no assumption of a linear model and they are particularly useful when the predictors may be associated in some non-linear fashion. One of the most fundamental differences between a decision tree and the linear model-type classifiers is the way in which splits are determined. Most classifiers involve the construction of predictor weights that often have a biological interpretation forced on to them. In effect they are interpreted as regression-type coefficients that describe the expected change in a response value, class in a classifier, as the predictor's value changes. The decision tree is different because the decisions involve thresholds rather than gradients. While this can be an advantage there are circumstances when it is not. If there is an obvious linear function the tree will require many nodes to build a stepped approximation to the function. This is illustrated in Figure 6.7.

Another important difference, for most decision trees, relates to the reuse of predictors. Predictors are never removed from consideration. This has several consequences. Firstly, there is no restriction on the number of linear splits as there is in a discriminant analysis, where the maximum number is the number of predictors or one less than the number of classes. Secondly, because a predictor can be reused in different nodes with different threshold values, it is possible for a predictor to have a context-dependent role in class determination.

The advantages of the decision tree approach can be summarised in nine points:

1. They learn by induction (generalising from examples) so there is no requirement for a pre-specified model. However, induction does not guarantee to find the correct tree.
2. Unlike the classifiers that use maximum likelihood methods to estimate parameter values, no single dominant data structure (e.g. normality) is assumed or required.
3. They are non-parametric because they do not require specification of a functional form for the relationship or the variable probability distributions (e.g. a general linear model).
4. Predictor selection algorithms are not needed because a robust stepwise selection method is used that never removes any variables.
5. The predictors do not require transforming to satisfy probability distribution constraints. The decision tree is invariant to monotonic predictor transformations (any transformation that retains the rank order of the cases), for example a logarithmic transformation will result in the same splits as the untransformed predictor.
6. Variables can be reused in different parts of a tree. This means that any context dependency of the predictors is automatically recognised. For example, the amount of soil phosphorus could be an important predictor, but only if the amount of soil nitrogen is above a certain threshold.
7. They are robust to the effects of outliers because the outliers can be isolated in their own nodes, which means that they have no effect on other cases.

8.   A mix of predictor data types can be used in some trees.
9.   Missing values may be handled by using surrogate variables.

The details behind the algorithms are described in the following sections. These sections explain how node purity is measured, how the best splits are identified, how tree complexity is determined and how missing values can be handled. For more detailed information Murthy (1998) is a useful survey of the algorithms used in decision trees.

Node purity

Decision trees attempt to divide the predictor space into homogeneous regions or terminal nodes, which contain examples from only one class. If it is impossible to produce an absolute separation of the classes, because either the predictors or the stopping rules prevent it, the goal changes to one of minimising the impurity of the nodes. Several algorithms are used to quantify this impurity. Some measure goodness instead of impurity, the difference being that a goodness value is maximised by the tree while impurity is minimised. Two of the most common measures are the Twoing Rule (a goodness measure) and the Gini Index (an impurity measure). The Twoing Rule (Breiman $et\ al.$, 1984) is defined as:

$$\text{Value} = (N_L/n).(N_R/n).(\Sigma|\,L_i/N_L - R_i/N_R|)^2$$

where N_L and N_R are the number of cases on the left and right sides of a split at node N, n is the number of cases at node N, and L_i and R_i are the number of cases in class i on the left and right of the split.

The Gini Index, which was originally a measure of the probability of misclassification, was proposed for decision trees by Breiman $et\ al.$ (1984). It has a value of zero when a node is pure, i.e. only contains cases from one class. It is defined as:

$$\text{Value} = 1 - (\text{class}_1/n)^2 - (\text{class}_2/n)^2$$

where class_1 is the number of class 1 cases in the left node, class_2 is the number of class 2 cases in the right node and n is the number of cases in the node.

Identifying splits

This is a computationally intensive activity. The most commonly used approach is an exhaustive search in which all possible splits, across all of the predictors, must be examined (Hand, 1997). For example, in the case of a continuous predictor the candidate splits are any values lying between actual predictor values. Apart from the computational overheads another disadvantage of this approach is that it tends to favour the predictors which have more potential splits. A computationally more efficient method, which also has less bias, uses a quadratic discriminant analysis to find the best split. This algorithm is at the centre of the QUEST decision tree (Loh and Shih, 1997). Irrespective of the algorithm used to find the splits the candidate splits have to be ranked with respect to their 'quality' so that the best can be selected. Different quality indicators are used, including the purity and goodness criteria described in the previous section. In addition other indices such as F values from an analysis of variance or variance reduction measures are used. Once the best split has been identified the data are partitioned according to the criterion and each partition must be examined to find its best split. Although this process could continue until each node was pure, it is not generally desirable. Instead the tree must be restricted by either halting its growth or pruning back from its maximum extent.

If a predictor variable is categorical, for example gender, a split based on each of the categories must be tried. This is relatively simple for a binary tree but can become very time consuming if the class has more than two categories.

Tree complexity

The structure of a decision tree reflects the characteristics of the training data, and any anomalies in the training data, due to noise or outliers, are likely to increase its complexity while reducing its future performance. In order to overcome these difficulties tree pruning methods are used to avoid trees with unreliable branches. This has the twin consequences of producing a tree that generates classifications more quickly and, more importantly, is better able to classify correctly independent test data. There are two approaches to pruning which depend on the timing. If pre-pruning, or a stopping rule, is used the tree is 'pruned' by halting its construction when some rule is triggered. At its simplest this could be a rule such that nodes can only be split if they have at least 100 cases. The obvious danger with this approach is that it stops too soon. Post-pruning is generally thought to be the best approach. The tree is allowed to grow to its maximum possible size and then branches are removed (pruned) until some criterion, such as acceptable classification accuracy, is reached.

The most common pruning technique makes use of cross-validation (Efron and Tibshirani, 1993), although a similar method can make use of a single separate test set of data. The cross-validation method begins by growing a large reference tree (no pruning) using all of the available data. This tree will have the maximum possible accuracy with the training data. However, the results from the cross-validated trees will be used to prune back this reference tree at the end of the exercise. Normally the data are split into ten folds for the cross-validation.

Each fold is withheld, in turn, from the data used to generate a decision tree. The unpruned decision trees generated from the remaining nine folds are tested on the withheld fold. This allows a comparison to be made between tree complexity and prediction accuracy with the withheld data. The classification error rates for the cross-validated trees, as a function of tree size, are averaged. Normally the relationship between cross-validated accuracy and tree size (number of nodes) will show that large trees have relatively poorer performance and that the best performance is found using smaller trees. The results of the cross-validation can be used to find the optimum tree size which is created by pruning back the original reference tree. The pruning of the reference tree is done iteratively, removing the least important nodes during each pruning cycle. The structures of the cross-validated trees, which will almost certainly differ from each other and the reference tree, are not considered; the only function for these trees is to find the optimum size for the reference tree.

Assigning classes to terminal nodes

When all of the cases in a terminal node share the same class the allocation of a class to the node is trivial. However, it is common to have terminal nodes with mixed classes. In such cases a rule is needed that decides on a class identity. The simplest rule is a majority vote in which the assigned class is the one with the most cases, albeit with some additional rule to deal with ties. The allocation of class labels becomes a little more complex if prior probabilities or costs are taken into account. Misclassification costs are described in more detail in the next chapter but they make allowances for the inequality of mislabelled classes. For example, labelling a malignant sample as benign is a more expensive mistake than the reverse. Once costs are included the aim of the classifier becomes one of minimising costs rather than errors. This can affect the structure of the tree by altering threshold values to favour the most expensive class and it can affect the allocation of class labels by effectively weighting the cases. This means that cases in the terminal node may be assigned to a minority class because this is the least expensive outcome. If an algorithm does not explicitly incorporate costs it is sometimes possible to alter the class prior probabilities so that the decision tree favours class allocations to the most expensive class.

Missing values

If a predictor value is missing, for example a sample recording failed, it may be impossible to apply a rule to the case. Most decision tree programs deal with this problem by using a sophisticated technique involving surrogate variables. This method uses the values from non-missing variables to estimate the missing value. For example, if two predictors, such as height and weight, are highly correlated it may be possible to obtain a reasonable estimate of a missing weight value from the height of a case. The implementation of surrogate variables is more sophisticated than a simple correlation and does not assume that surrogates are global, instead they are adjusted depending on the identity of the cases in the node. Usually, the selected surrogate variable is the one which generates a split of the current node that is the most similar to that achieved using the original variable.

6.2.2   Example analysis

This example analyses the cancer data from Section 5.4.3 using the classification and regression trees algorithm (Breiman *et al.*, 1984) from SPSS AnswerTree 3.0. This method generates binary decision trees by splitting data subsets, using all predictor variables, to create two child nodes. The best predictor was chosen using the Gini impurity measure to produce data partitions which were as homogeneous as possible with respect to the cancer class. Ten-fold cross-validation was used to obtain the appropriately sized tree. Two analyses are described that differ only in the misclassification costs. In the first analysis equal misclassification costs were applied. This means that classifying a malignant sample as benign is assumed to carry the same cost as classifying a benign sample as malignant. In the second analysis classifying a malignant sample as benign was assumed to be five times more costly than classifying a benign sample as malignant.

The tree with misclassification costs is a subset of the equal cost tree. Figure 6.3 shows the tree for unequal misclassification costs and Figure 6.4 shows the additional nodes added to the previous tree when costs were equal. Only four of the predictors were used, some more than once. The initial split is a very simple and powerful filter that uses the uniformity of cell size at a threshold of 2.5. If this is combined with a test on the bare nuclei only 5 out 239 (2.1%) malignant samples are misclassified. This is further reduced to 2 (0.7%) if clump thickness is also included.

Misclassification costs surprisingly come into play on the right-hand side of the tree. It is surprising because the first node on this side of the tree (node 2) contains mainly malignant samples. If there were no more splits below node 2 there would be no misclassified malignant cases on this side of the tree but 38 false positives (8.6% of all benign samples). What happens to this side of the tree depends on the misclassification costs. If they are equal a more complex tree is produced with additional splits below node 6 (Figure 6.4). This results in five false negatives (malignant samples identified as benign) and ten false negatives. If false positives are given a cost that is five times larger than the false negatives the tree

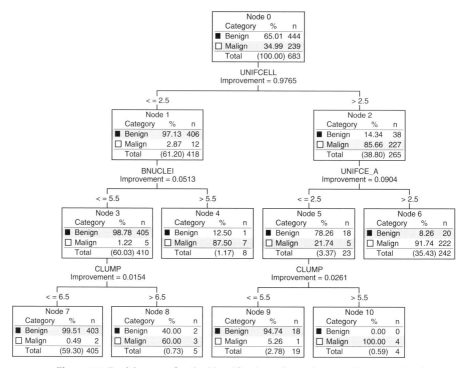

Figure 6.3 Decision tree for the identification of samples as malignant or benign. This tree uses unequal misclassification costs for the two classes. Predictors are: UNIFCELL, uniformity of cell size; CLUMP, clump thickness; UNIFCE_A, uniformity of cell shape; BNUCLEI, bare nuclei.

halts at node 6 with one false negative and twenty false positives. This is because the false positives are sacrificed to 'protect' the more expensive misidentification. This means that, overall, the cost-sensitive tree makes more mistakes but at a reduced cost.

6.2.3   *Random forests*

As with all other classifiers, decision trees have their problems. In particular, they can be less accurate than methods such as support vector machines and the structure of the trees can be unstable (Breiman, 1996). The instability is often seen when small changes to the training data produce significant changes to the tree, either in the identity of the split variables or the value for the split. Despite these changes to the structure the accuracy may be affected much less. Breiman and Cutler (2004a) noted that if you 'change the data a little you get a different picture. So the interpretation of what goes on is built on shifting sands'. Breiman (2001a,b) developed an algorithm, called

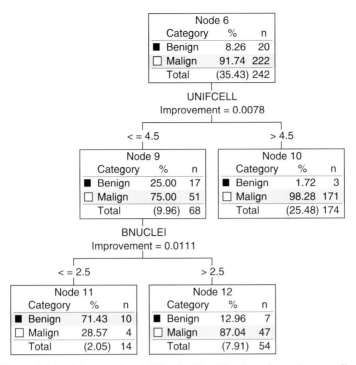

Figure 6.4 Decision tree (partial) for the identification of samples as malignant or benign. This tree uses equal misclassification costs for the two classes. This tree is identical to that of Figure 6.3 except for the additional splits below node 6.

RandomForests (a trademark of Salford Systems), that is said to overcome many of these shortcomings while retaining, and possibly enhancing, their interpretability. RandomForest classifiers performed well in the comparisons made by Lee *et al.* (2005), in which they consistently outperformed other decision trees and many other methods. Breiman and Cutler (2004b) listed some of the important features of RandomForests:

- They have an accuracy that equals or exceeds many current classifiers and they cannot overfit.
- They are efficient (fast) on large databases and can handle thousands of predictors without selection routines.
- They estimate the importance of each predictor.
- They generate an unbiased estimate of the generalisation error.
- They have robust algorithms to deal with missing data and for balancing the error if class proportions are markedly different.
- They compute the proximities between pairs of cases that can be used in clustering and identifying outliers.

- There is an experimental method for detecting variable interactions.
- Generated forests can be saved for future use on other data.

The algorithm generates many trees, the forest, and each tree in the forest differs with respect to the makeup of its training cases and the predictors used at each node. Each training set is a bootstrapped sample, with n equal to the original sample size, from the original data. The number of predictors for each node in a tree (m) is set to be much less than the total available. A set of m predictors is drawn, at random, from those available for each node in the tree. This means that the predictors considered for the splits are unlikely to be the same for any node in the tree. The value of m, which is the only adjustable parameter to which random forests are sensitive (Breiman and Cutler, 2004a), is the same for all trees in the forest. No pruning is used, instead each tree is grown to the largest extent possible. Growing trees to their maximum extent helps to keep the bias low.

Breiman (2001a) showed that the forest error rate depends on two things. First, and unsurprisingly, increasing the strength (accuracy) of the individual trees decreases the forest error rate. Second, and less obviously, there may be a correlation between pairs of trees. As pairs of trees become more correlated the forest error rate increases. Reducing m, the number of predictors, reduces both the correlation and the strength. It is therefore important to find the optimum value for m so that the correlation is reduced but without too much effect on the strength of the trees. Fortunately it seems that the optimal range for m is usually quite wide and an out-of-bag error rate can be used to find an appropriate value.

Each tree is built from a bootstrapped sample that typically contains about two-thirds of the cases. The remaining third, the out-of-bag sample, is run through the finished tree. Some trees will correctly predict the class of these cases others will not. The proportion of times that a case is misclassified, averaged over all cases, is the out-of-bag error rate. The out-of-bag error rate is also part of the recommended way of deciding on an appropriate value for m (Breiman and Cutler, 2004a). They suggest starting with a value for m that is the square root of the total number of predictors. About 25 trees should be run with increasing and decreasing values of m until the minimum out-of-bag error is obtained.

RandomForests have other advantages apart from increased prediction accuracy. They can also be used to estimate the importance of each variable and the associations between cases. In order to estimate the importance of predictor p its values in the ith tree are permuted randomly among all of the out-of-bag cases. This is a similar approach to that used in the Mantel test. The raw importance score for predictor p is the difference in accuracy between the tree with the unaltered, and the permutated values, of p. If this is repeated for all predictors across all trees it is possible to obtain a z-score for each predictor from its mean raw importance score divided the standard error of the raw importance scores. The z-scores can then be used to rank the predictors, with the most important predictors having the largest z-scores. A different measure, which appears to yield similar results, is the sum of the Gini Index which decreases each time that a predictor is used to split a node.

The association, or proximity, between cases can be found from the number of times that they occur together in the same terminal node. These counts are normalised by dividing by the number of trees, producing a proximity matrix that can be analysed using a metric scaling method (Section 2.6). Apart from showing the proximity of cases these distance matrices and their metrically scaled projections can be used to replace missing values, locate outliers and investigate how the predictors separate the classes by locating 'prototypes'. A prototype definition for class i begins by finding the case which has largest number of class i cases among its k nearest neighbours. The medians of the values for these cases, across all predictors, are the medians for the class i prototype. The upper and lower quartiles for these neighbours also provide evidence for the stability of the prototype medians. The procedure can be repeated to find additional class prototypes, but with a constraint such that the cases in the previous neighbourhood are not considered.

Liaw and Wiener (2006) have written an R function that is based on the original Fortran program written by Breiman and Cutler. In addition to the usual R manual pages it is worth consulting Breiman's (2002) notes on running the original program. The following simple example is taken from the manual for the R randomForest function (Version 4.5-16) and uses Fisher's *Iris* data (Section 2.10). Five hundred random trees were grown with two predictors tested at each split. The out-of-bag error rate was 5.33% (eight cases), made up of three *versicolor* mislabelled as *virginica* and five *virginica* mislabelled as *versicolor*. While this is about the best that any classifier can achieve with these data the analysis provides the extra information about variable importance (Table 6.1). It is clear that the two petal measurements are much more important than the sepal measurements, with the same rank order across all measures: petal width > petal length > sepal length > sepal width.

The MDS plot (Figure 6.5) echoes all of the previous analyses with *I. setosa* clearly separated from the other two species. It is important to remember that this plot uses distances based on case proximities in terminal nodes rather than actual floral measurements. The class prototypes, based on these 150 observations, are shown in Figure 6.6 and Table 6.2.

Table 6.1. *Importance statistics for the four predictors*

Predictor	*I. setosa*	*I. versicolor*	*I. virginica*	Mean decrease in accuracy	Mean decrease in the Gini index
Sepal length	1.15	1.99	1.69	1.36	8.12
Sepal width	0.97	−0.14	0.86	0.51	2.49
Petal length	3.73	4.44	4.23	2.51	42.68
Petal width	3.75	4.47	4.35	2.51	46.00

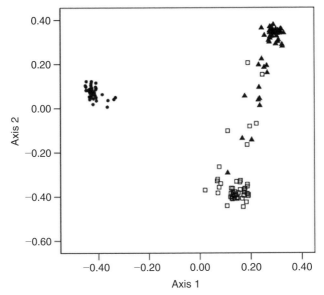

Figure 6.5 Multidimensional scaling plot of the between-cases proximities from 500 trees. *I. setosa*; filled circles; *I. versicolor*; open squares; *I. virginica*; filled triangles.

Despite its many advantages RandomForests do not appear to have been widely used in biological applications, possibly because it is such a recent technique. Lee *et al.* (2005) used the method in a series of comparative tests on various microarray data sets and it performed well. Cummings and Myers (2004) found that RandomForests had the greatest accuracy in predicting C-to-U edited sites while Segal *et al.* (2004) included RandomForests as one method used to relate HIV-1 sequence variation to replication capacity. Prasad *et al.* (2006) recommended RandomForests, and other bagging and boosting methods, as a suitable approach for predictive mapping.

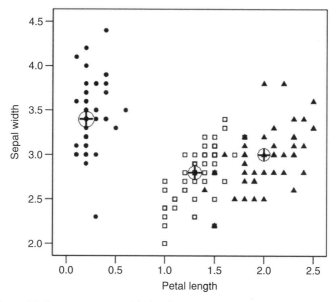

Figure 6.6 Prototype centres (circle with cross) overlaid on a plot of sepal length against petal width. Symbols are the same as in Figure 6.5.

Table 6.2. *Class prototype values for the three* Iris *species*

Species	Sepal length	Sepal width	Petal length	Petal width
I. setosa	5.00	3.4	1.5	0.2
I. versicolor	5.85	2.8	4.3	1.3
I. virginica	6.50	3.0	5.6	2.0

6.2.4   Other 'flavours'

There are many other 'flavours' of decision tree that differ largely in the rules used to generate the splits and the allowable data types. Four of the more common algorithms are described briefly in this section.

ID3, C4.5 and C5

The ID3 (iterative dichotomising 3rd algorithm) was published by Quinlan in 1979 and evolved into the C4.5 and C5 algorithms. All three algorithms feature prominently in artificial intelligence and machine learning studies but are rarely encountered in biological research. These algorithms use information gain criteria to select predictors for the splits. Information gain is not explained in detail here but it is related to the diversity indices with which most ecologists will be familiar. For example, the entropy of a predictor is given by $E = \Sigma(-p-p_i.\log_2 p_i)$, where p_i is the proportion of cases in class i. For example, if there are 40 cases made up of 18 males and 22 females the entropy for gender would be $-(18/40).\log_2(18/40) + (22/40).\log_2(22/40)$ or 0.993. This value is close 1.0 which would indicate that the predictor contains little information. A value of zero arises when all the cases are in one class. If the frequencies had been 5 and 35 the entropy value would be 0.543.

Suppose that 8 of the 18 males and 20 of the 22 females are from class one, meaning that 10 males and 2 females are in class two. If gender was used as a split the resulting nodes would have 8 class one and 2 class two cases in the male node and 20 class one and 10 class two cases in the female node. The information gain, which is the difference in entropy before and after considering gender as a splitting variable, would be:

$$\text{Gain}(\text{class, gender}) = E(\text{gender}) - (10/18. E(\text{gender} = \text{male}))$$

$$- (20/22. E(\text{gender} = \text{female}))$$

$$\text{Gain}(\text{class, gender}) = 0.993 - (0.555.0.991) - (0.909.0.439)$$

$$\text{Gain}(\text{class, gender}) = 0.048$$

Once the gain has been calculated for each predictor the one with the largest value is chosen to split the node. Unlike most other decision trees a predictor can only be used once. If gender was selected to split the first node it could not be used further down the tree.

Because of some of the limitations of the ID3 algorithm Quinlan developed the C4.5 and C5 algorithms. C4.5 uses continuously valued predictors by employing a local discretisation algorithm that adjusts the categories for each node. The other important improvements were the addition of tree pruning algorithms to improve its performance with novel data and the incorporation of misclassification costs. Quinlan's web page, and the source for the commercial implementation of the C5 algorithm, is http://www.rulequest.com/.

CHAID

The CHAID (chi-square automatic interaction detection) algorithm is another of the older decision tree algorithms and was devised by Kass (1980) as a more robust form of the earlier AID algorithm. It is restricted to categorical predictors, although continuous predictors can be used by first converting them into a small number of ordinal, discrete categories. Splits are based on the magnitude of a chi-square statistic from a cross tabulation of class against predictor categories. The CHAID algorithm reduces the number of predictor categories by merging categories when there is no significant difference between them with respect to the class. When no more classes can be merged the predictor can be considered as a candidate for a split at the node. The original CHAID algorithm is not guaranteed to find the best (most significant) split of all of those examined because it uses the last split tested. The Exhaustive CHAID algorithm attempts to overcome this problem by continuing to merge categories, irrespective of significance levels, until only two categories remain for each predictor. It then uses the split with the largest significance value rather than the last one tried.

The CHAID algorithm treats missing values as another predictor class, for example gender could have three classes: male, female and unknown. It is possible that a split at a node could be based on a missing value.

QUEST

The QUEST algorithm (quick, unbiased, efficient, statistical tree) has been shown to be one of the best classifiers in comparison with others (Lim *et al.*, 2000) and it has been incorporated into a number of commercial packages, including SPSS AnswerTree (see Figure 6.3). Details of the algorithm are given in Loh and Shih (1997) and the program can be downloaded from http://www.stat.wisc.edu/~loh. QUEST has been shown to be very fast: in one test Loh and Shih (1997) report that QUEST completed one analysis in 1 CPU second compared with 30.5 hours for an alternative algorithm. It also has negligible variable selection bias, which is achieved by using a variety of significance tests such as *F*- and chi-squared tests to select the predictor and then employing cluster and quadratic discriminant analyses on the selected variable to find a split point.

OC1

Decision trees that work with single variables produce splits (hyperplanes) that are parallel to one of the predictor axes (Figure 6.2). If the splits are linear combinations of one or more predictors the hyperplanes can be both oblique and parallel. Figure 6.7 is an example where a tree built using univariate splits is complex and non-intuitive, essentially building a stepped function along the diagonal, while a multivariate split could be achieved with a single node (if $(x-y) \geq 0$ then class $= 1$ else class $= 2$). Although the use of a multivariate linear combination significantly reduces the tree complexity it usually comes with the disadvantage that ease of interpretation has been sacrificed. OC1 (oblique classifier 1; Murthy *et al.*, 1994) is a decision tree that is capable of producing oblique hyperplanes from numeric (continuous) predictor values. Although the splits are multivariate rather than univariate Murthy *et al.* (1994) prefer to refer to the splits as oblique rather than multivariate because the latter term includes

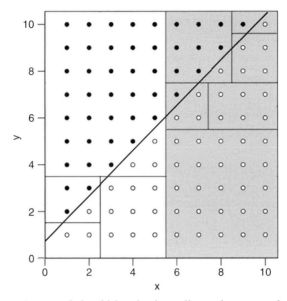

Figure 6.7 An example in which univariate splits produce a complex tree but a single multivariate split $(x - y \geq 0$, diagonal line) will produce complete separation. The splits were created by the classification and regression tree from SPSS AnswerTree 3.0 algorithm (not all splits are shown). The shaded area highlights the regions separated by the first split.

non-linear combinations of predictors that would produce curved surfaces. OC1 was recently used as part of a system to predict gene models (Allen *et al.*, 2004). OC1 can be obtained from http://www.cs.jhu.edu/~salzberg/announce-oc1.html.

6.3   Support vector machines

Support vector machines (SVMs) are one of the most recently developed classifiers and build on developments in computational learning theory. They are attracting attention, particularly in bioinformatic applications, because of their accuracy and their ability to deal with a large number of predictors, indeed they appear to be relatively immune to the 'curse of dimensionality'. Unfortunately, descriptions and explanations of SVMs are heavily mathematical and the following explanation is a considerable over-simplification. More detail is provided by Burges (1998). This is an excellent tutorial which uses the VC dimension as a starting point and presents proofs of most of the main theorems. There is a less mathematical description of SVMs in Burbidge *et al.* (2001) who show that a SVM outperforms a neural network and decision tree in a structure−activity problem related to drug design. DTREG is a commercial classification and regression tree program and its website a very clear graphical explanation of the SVM algorithm (http://www.dtreg.com/svm.htm).

Most of the previous classifiers separate classes using hyperplanes that split the classes, using a flat plane, within the predictor space. Unfortunately, in many non-trivial problems, a perfect linear separator does not exist. SVMs extend the concept of hyperplane separation to data that cannot be separated linearly, by mapping the predictors onto a new, higher-dimensional space (called the feature space) in which they can be separated linearly (Figure 6.8). Although it is possible to separate the classes in any training set, given a sufficiently large feature space, this incurs computational and mathematical costs, while simultaneously running the risk of finding trivial solutions that over-fit the data. Consequently, the SVM algorithm includes methods that aim to avoid this over-fitting. This is achieved by using an iterative optimisation algorithm which seeks to minimise an error function. The error function is not a simple count of the incorrectly classified cases, instead it incorporates a user-defined constant that penalises the amount of error in class allocations. In general, these misclassifications should only arise if the wrong kernel function has been selected or there are cases in different classes (possibly mislabelled) which have the same predictor vectors. If the constant is set to a high value it could result in a classifier that performs well with training data but poorly with new data.

The method's name derives from the support vectors, which are lists of the predictor values obtained from cases that lie closest to the decision boundary separating the classes and are, therefore, potentially the most difficult to classify. It is reasonable to assume that these cases have the greatest impact on the location of the decision boundary. Indeed, if they were removed they could have large effects on its location. Computationally, finding the best location for the decision plane is an optimisation problem that makes uses of a kernel function to

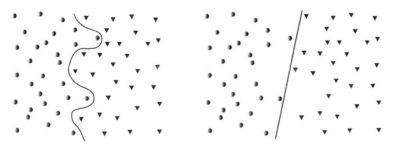

Figure 6.8 Diagrammatic representation of the hypothetical decision boundaries for two classes in the original (left) predictor space and transformed (right) feature space.

construct linear boundaries through non-linear transformations, or mappings, of the predictors. The 'clever' part of the algorithm is that it finds a hyperplane in the predictor space which is stated in terms of the input vectors and dot products in the feature space. A dot product is the cosine of the angle between two vectors (lists of predictor values) that have normalised lengths. The dot product can then be used to find the distances between the vectors in this higher dimensional space. A SVM locates the hyperplane that separates the support vectors without ever representing the space explicitly. Instead a kernel function is used that plays the role of the dot product in the feature space.

Figure 6.8 is a diagrammatic simplification of the process. The two classes can only be separated completely by a complex curve in the original space of the predictor. The best linear separator cannot completely separate the two classes. However, if the original predictor values can be projected into a more suitable 'feature space' it is possible to separate completely the classes with a linear decision boundary. Consequently, the problem becomes one of finding the appropriate transformation.

The kernel function, which is central to the SVM approach, is also one of the biggest problems, particularly with respect to the selection of its parameter values. It is also necessary to select the magnitude of the penalty for violating the soft margin between the classes. This means that successful construction of a SVM requires some decisions that should be informed by the data to be classified. Finally, they can also be relatively slow because of their algorithmic complexity. Despite these problems the SVM approach has shown great promise and there are quite a large number of examples of their use to classify sample types using microarray data. For example, Brown *et al.* (2000) tested SVMs with microarray data and used one to predict functional roles for uncharacterised yeast ORFs based on their expression data and Furey *et al.* (2000) used one to identify a mislabelled case before completely separating two classes. Rogers *et al.* (2005) is a survey of class prediction methods using microarray data and uses a SVM in an example analysis.

6.4   Artificial neural networks

6.4.1   Introduction

When the field of artificial intelligence (AI) was founded in 1956 it was generally believed that machines could be made to simulate intelligent behaviour, and by the 1960s there were two main AI branches personified by two of the early pioneers. Minsky, at MIT, was concerned with a symbolic approach to AI. This symbolic, rule-based, approach is closely linked to expert systems and programming languages such as LISP and Prolog. Rosenblatt, whose origins were in psychology, used a connectionist approach to AI that was based on a simplified biological neural network. The early promise of the connectionist approach was almost fatally damaged by a highly critical evaluation of its limitations (Minsky and Papert, 1969). However, the connectionist approach was rejuvenated in the 1980s, particularly following the publication of McClelland and Rumelhart's (1986) influential book *Parallel Distributed Processing*.

Artificial neural networks belong to a class of methods variously known as parallel distributed processing or connectionist techniques. They are an attempt to simulate a real neural network, which is composed of a large number of interconnected, but independent, neurons. However, most artificial neural networks are simulated since they are implemented in software on a single CPU, rather than one CPU per neuron.

It is generally considered that neural networks do well when data structures are not well understood. This is because they are able to combine and transform raw data without any user input (Hand and Henley, 1997). Thus they are of particular value when, as is the case for many ecological examples, the problem is poorly understood. If there is considerable background knowledge, including knowledge of probability density distributions, it is usually better to use methods that incorporate this information (Hand and Henley, 1997).

It is probably safe to say that these methods have not delivered all that was originally expected of them. This failure to deliver fully is possibly a consequence of too much expectation combined with their frequent inappropriate use (see Schwarzer *et al.* (2000) for detailed examples). Many artificial neural networks replicate standard statistical methods, but with the added complication of a lack of transparency. In general, they perform well when the main requirement is for a 'black box' classifier rather than a classifier that provides insight into the nature of class differences.

Only a brief outline of the details is given below. There are many sources which provide detailed accounts of the algorithms or how neural networks relate to statistical techniques, such as generalised linear models. Six particular sources are recommended. Undoubtedly the most important book is Ripley's (1996) *Pattern Recognition and Neural Networks*. Boddy and Morris (1999) describe, amongst others, the background to multilayer perceptrons and radial bias function networks, set within the context of automated species identification. Cheng and Titterington (1994) and Sarle (1994) review the links between neural networks and statistical methods. Goodman and Harrell (2001a,b) provide very useful descriptions of multilayer perceptrons and their links to generalised linear modelling. The background to multilayer perceptrons is set in the context of their very powerful and free NEVPROP neural network software

(Goodman, 1996) that is used elsewhere in this section. Finally, there are the neural network FAQs at ftp://ftp.sas.com/pub/neural/FAQ.html. These FAQs were last updated in 2002.

6.4.2   Back-propagation networks

An artificial neural network is composed of a number of relatively simple processing elements called nodes or neurons. A node converts a weighted sum of inputs to a bounded (0−1) output value. The conversion of the weighted sum to the output is carried out by a transfer function that is typically sigmoidal, for example the logistic function in which the output is $1/(1 + e^{-input})$, where the input is $\Sigma w_i.p_i +$ constant. In neural network terminology the constant is known as the bias. The structure of a single node is summarised in Figure 6.9. Although there is only one processing node in Figure 6.9 the resulting network is equivalent to the logistic generalised linear model (GLM) described in the previous chapter.

The power, and problems, of neural networks comes from having a network with more than one node, possibly arranged in interconnected layers. The number of inputs will be fixed by the number of predictors and the number of outputs is fixed by the number of classes. Only one output is required for two classes. However, there is great potential for flexibility between the input and output layers. A typical neural network, although there are many other architectures, would have three layers: input; hidden (middle); and output. The example shown in Figure 6.10 also has a skip-layer connection for one of the inputs. This type of network is known as a multi-layer perceptron. The network

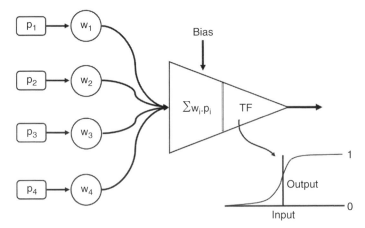

Figure 6.9 Structure of a stylised neural network node. w_i are the weights connecting the predictor (p_i) values to the node which uses a logistic transfer function (shown at the lower right).

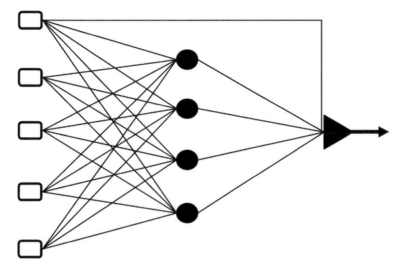

Figure 6.10 Generalised artificial neural network with three layers. The input layer (open boxes) has five nodes that are fully interconnected to four nodes (filled circles) in a hidden layer that are, in turn, connected to a single output (triangle) node. In addition, the first input node has a direct, skip-layer, connection to the output node.

in Figure 6.10 has 25 weights: four from each of the five input nodes to the hidden layer; four from the hidden layer to the output node; and one on the skip-layer connection. Because of this complexity it is probable that the network would be reasonably tolerant of missing values. It also means that the network's model of the relationship between the predictors and the class (the output) is dispersed, or distributed, through its weights. Unfortunately, the distribution of the learned relationship, amongst the weights, makes them difficult to interpret.

The problem that must be solved is finding appropriate values for these weights to maximise the accuracy of the predictions given a set of training data. This is achieved via a series of iterative adjustments to the weights during a training phase. One of the most common algorithms used to implement this training is known as back-propagation although there are others such as the Levenberg–Marquardt algorithm and conjugate gradient descent.

The network begins with randomised values for the weights. At this point there is no reason to believe that the network will perform any better than chance. The first case is presented to the network and its inputs pass through the 25 weights and five transfer functions to produce a real-valued output within the range 0–1. In a simple two-class problem the two classes would have the values 0 and 1. If a simple threshold is applied the case will have a predicted class of 0 if the output is less than 0.5 and class 1 if the output is greater than 0.5.

Any difference between the actual class and the output is a measure of network's current inaccuracy which is due to inappropriate weights. The error can be corrected if the weights are adjusted. The problem is deciding which weights to adjust since they may differ in their contributions to the prediction error. It is also reasonable to assume that the magnitude of the adjustment should take account of the size of the error. If the error is small only small weight adjustments are required. The back-propagation weight correction algorithm measures how the error is propagated back through the network's weights. After the weights have been adjusted the next case is applied to the network and the weight adjustment procedure is repeated. Once all of the cases in the training set have passed through the network one epoch has been completed. The entire training cycle may require hundreds of epochs, the end point being determined by some pre-specified termination criterion such as a minimum error rate.

The rule by which individual weights are adjusted takes account of the size of the output error and the magnitudes of the outputs from the nodes feeding directly, or indirectly, into the output node. If it is assumed that nodes with the largest outputs make the largest contribution to the output error then their weights should experience the largest changes. The mathematical details and proofs are widely available and are not given here. However, a simplified version is that the change in weight for a node is equal to its error multiplied by its output. The weight changes are moderated by a learning rate that alters the rate of change. This is needed to avoid a situation in which weights oscillate either side of their optimum values. In order to minimise training times, whilst also avoiding the trap of becoming stuck in a local minimum, a momentum term is also applied. The momentum takes account of the magnitude of the previous weight change and adjusts the current weight change to take account of this by reinforcing changes that are in the same direction. Essentially, this accelerates the rate of change when it is appropriate.

Deciding when to stop training is important because if a network is over-trained its future performance will be compromised. Usually, a decision to halt training is based on the size of the training error that is measured as the sum of squared errors. In a statistical model there are well-defined rules that guarantee to find the parameter values that minimise the error. However, because network training is heuristic the rules do not exist and judgement has to be employed instead. In order to avoid over-fitting, part of the data is reserved for testing. If the network becomes over-trained the test error will begin to rise, even though the training error may still be declining. An increase in the testing error is an indication that training should stop. Ideally the network should experience a final test using a third set of data that played no part in the training.

6.4.3   *Modelling general and generalised linear models with neural networks*

Despite their biological inspiration many neural networks are really re-badged statistical techniques. Indeed Goodman (1996) refers to his NevProp neural network software as a multivariate non-linear regression program. As shown below many of the statistical classifiers can be duplicated by an appropriate network design. Goodman and Harrell (2001a,b) have proposed a formalised method for deciding if a neural network should be used in preference to a GLM. The only circumstances that they recommend a neural network over a GLM are when the relationships between the class and predictors involve both non-linear relationships and between-predictor interactions. In such circumstances it is probably more efficient to use a neural network. However, Goodman and Harrell (2001a,b) emphasise an important difference between the two approaches that extends across all of the classifiers described in this book. The statistical approach to classifiers tends to concentrate on the parameter values and their significance levels as a guide to the adequacy of the model. The wider machine learning approach, which certainly applies to neural networks, is less concerned with predictor values and more concerned with the classifier's accuracy when presented with novel data.

A number of network designs are described in this section and associated with specific statistical models. Most of these designs are then used, and compared, in Section 6.4.6. As shown in Figure 6.11, a simple network with one processing node is effectively a GLM. Each predictor is linked by a single weight, or coefficient, to the output node where a logistic transfer is applied to convert the weighted sum to an output within the range 0 to 1. When statistical models are built it is usual to investigate if various predictor transformations can improve the fit.

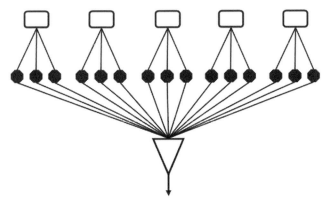

Figure 6.11 A 'transforming' neural network in which each predictor input has its own hidden layer of three nodes.

If a single hidden layer neural network is constructed, with fully connected links between the input nodes and the hidden nodes, the network can model, simultaneously, predictor transformations and interactions. The complexity of these transformations and interactions is controlled by the size of the hidden layer. Goodman and Harrell (2001a,b) suggest two parallel analyses, following on from suitable exploratory analyses, which compare the results from a generalised model with those of a neural network with a single hidden layer. The GLM should not include any interactions or predictor transformations. The comparisons between the two classifiers should include the AUC of a ROC plot (Section 7.7) and Nagelkerke's R^2. If the predictive accuracy of this network is not significantly better than the GLM there are two conclusions. Firstly, there is no point using a neural network and, secondly, there is no need to consider incorporating interactions or predictor transformations into another iteration of the GLM. If there had been important interactions or required transformations the network's accuracy would have been superior.

If the network's accuracy was significantly better there must have been interactions and/or transformations missing from the GLM. The next step recommended by Goodman and Harrell (2001a,b) depends on the data types of the predictors. If all of the predictors were binary the network's improvement was due to interactions and it is probably worth continuing to use the network or spend time trying to identify the important interactions for inclusion in the GLM. However, if the predictors are non-binary it is necessary to isolate inter-action improvements from those created by transformations. This can be achieved by creating a neural network that cannot model interactions but can transform the predictors automatically. A transforming network has a hidden layer in which groups of hidden nodes are connected to only one of the inputs (Figure 6.11). This hidden layer, made up of node clusters, performs the necessary transformations, without a need to specify a functional form. As the size of the transforming layer is increased the transformations can become arbitrarily complex and serve a similar function to the smoothing function in a generalised additive model (GAM) (Section 5.6). If this transforming network performs as well as the original network the improvement was due to transformations rather than interactions. It is probably worthwhile finding suitable transforma-tions to include in a GLM. However, if the transforming network is not as accurate as the original network it is worth considering using a neural network.

A GAM can be fully simulated by adding a second hidden layer. For example, using the network in Figure 6.11, each set of transforming nodes would be connected to only one of five nodes in the second layer. These are then connected to the output. In this way each predictor is subjected to a smoothing function before feeding in a GLM (the second hidden layer plus the output).

Although these comparisons may sound like a very time-consuming process, Goodman and Harrell (2001a,b) point out that using neural networks in this exploratory role avoids the need to spend time trying to refine a GLM when it is not needed or possibly too complex. It also provides a solid case for the use of a neural network when it is justified.

6.4.4   Interpreting weights

One of the most important disadvantages that is often cited for neural networks is that they are black boxes. Even if they are accurate it is difficult to understand the relationship between the predictors and the class. The problem is that a predictor's contribution can be spread across several nodes and layers. The interpretation is further complicated by the non-uniqueness of a particular weight matrix. For example, changing the order in which cases are presented to the network, or the values for the initial weights, will probably alter the final weight distribution, even if it has no effect on the accuracy. Consequently, there are no simple rules for directly interpreting the weights.

Intrator and Intrator (2001) and Goodman (1996) both describe methods that allow some interpretation of the contribution made by each predictor to the outcome. Both methods make use of the fact that, in a back-propagation network, a predictor's generalised weights have the same interpretation as the weights in a logistic regression (Section 5.4), i.e. their contribution to the log odds. If a predictor could have a positive effect for some cases, and a negative effect for others, it could lead to a mean effect of zero, but with a large variance. A small variance in the generalised weights would arise when a predictor's effect was consistent suggesting a linear relationship (Intrator and Intrator, 2001), while a large variance is suggestive of a non-linear effect. Details of the algorithms are not given here but both use repeated simulations to explore the variability in weights. Intrator and Intrator (2001) stress that weight interpretation, using their method, is only possible if a skip-layer architecture is used. This means that, in addition to any hidden layer connections, there is a direct connection between the predictor inputs and the output layer. Goodman and Harrell (2001a) also recommend these skip-layer connections because they represent direct linear effects of the predictors and they tend to add stability to the network whilst also decreasing the time needed to train the network. Goodman's NevProp software also includes an option to apply a Bayesian method called automatic relevance detection to rank the predictors by their importance to the network.

Geverey *et al.* (2003) and Olden *et al.* (2004) are empirical tests of a range of weight interpretation algorithms. Geverey *et al.* (2003) used a 'real' data set while Olden *et al.* (2004) applied the methods to an artificial data set whose structure was known. Olden *et al.* (2004) compared the ranked predictor importance across the weight interpretation algorithms and their correspondence to the real structure of the data. They concluded that one of the simplest methods, the connection weight approach, was the best. This approach is illustrated in the worked example (Section 6.4.6) and compared with the automatic relevance detection rankings from NevProp.

6.4.5   Radial bias function networks

Although it may not be immediately apparent a multilayer perceptron neural network constructs hyperplanes to divide up the predictor space between the classes. It is also possible to divide up space using spheres, or hyperspheres as they are known when there are more than three dimensions. At its simplest a hypersphere is described by its centre and radius. However, it is more useful if the hypersphere takes account of the position of cases within the sphere, in particular their distance from the centre. This is possible if the sphere, or kernel as it is more generally known, is described by function such as the Gaussian (normal distribution). A network constructed to use hyperspheres instead of hyperplanes is known as a radial basis function (RBF) network. RBF networks have a number of advantages over multilayer perceptrons and they have proven to be very successful at species identification tasks (see Boddy and Morris (1999) for examples). Their first advantage is that some of the design decisions are removed because they can model any non-linear function using a single hidden layer. However, there are other important decisions, described below, that will affect the network's performance. Their second advantage is that they do not require the same amount of training because standard linear modelling techniques can be employed. In addition to being much faster the linear modelling methods are not heuristic and so they do not suffer from the local minima problems which can be a problem for multilayer perceptrons.

The data are generalised by kernels, or basis functions and the trick is to find the appropriate number, parameters and locations for them. The number of kernels is equal to the number of hidden layer nodes. The kernel centres are initially placed at random locations before their positions are adjusted using a variety of methods. For example, randomly selected cases from the training data could be used but sampling error may create problems if the hidden layer is small (only a small sample of points would be used). Alternatively, a method such as *k*-means clustering could be used to find the kernel centres and to place each case into a cluster. A Gaussian kernel is characterised by its location and its spread. The spread, or smoothing factor, must also be determined. If the spread is small the Gaussian kernels are very spiky and the network will interpolate poorly, resulting in poor generalisation. Alternatively, if the spread is too wide the detail may be lost. As a guideline the spread is usually selected so that each kernel overlaps a few centres of neighbouring kernels. Although the spread of a kernel can be user-defined they are usually determined by the data during one of the training passes. Generally, the kernels will not all have the same spread since smaller kernels are appropriate if there is a high density of points in one region.

The network is trained by only two passes through the training data. During these passes the kernel spreads and output layer weights are set. The output weights connect the hidden radial units to an output layer which is made up of standard nodes with linear transfer functions. The output from each kernel, for a particular case, is a function of the distance between the case and the kernel's centre. These outputs are processed by the output layer's weights and transfer functions to produce an output which determines the predicted class for a case.

Despite their undoubted advantage they have disadvantages. For example, RBF networks may not extrapolate well with novel data that is at, or beyond, the periphery of the training data. This is because this region of predictor space will be poorly represented by the kernels.

6.4.6   Example analysis

The cancer data set (Section 5.4.3) is analysed using Goodman's (1996) NevProp software. Apart from being freely available, NevProp also provides great flexibility in the design of the networks and comprehensive summary information about the analyses. Three network designs are tested and the results are compared with the logistic regression and GAM results from the previous chapter. The three designs are:

1.   No hidden layer — a GLM equivalent to logistic regression.
2.   A single, fully interconnected, hidden layer — a GLM that includes automatic detection of interactions and the application of suitable transformations.
3.   A single, clustered, transforming hidden layer (Figure 6.11) — a GLM equivalent to logistic regression but with automatic predictor transformation and no interactions.

The data were split into a training component (two-thirds or 454 cases) and a testing component (one-third, 228 cases). The testing component was withheld for final testing once the networks had been trained, i.e. these data played no part in the training of the networks. The networks were trained in two phases. In the first phase, five cross-validated splits of the training data were used to build networks in which the performance was assessed on the withheld segment of the training data. Five splits were used to reduce the variance in the error that always arises during cross-validated training. The cross-validated splits used 70% of the training data to estimate the weights while the accuracy was tested on the withheld 30% of the training data. In the second training phase the entire training set (484 cases) was used to fit a model. However, training halted when it reached the criteria established during the first training phase. Once the final network had been trained it was tested using the separate test set.

One of the difficulties in designing a neural network is ensuring that the network does not become too complex, i.e. too many weights, for the problem. NevProp has a non-linear extension of ridge regression, plus a hyper-parameter, that adjusts a penalty for groups of units, according to the number of well-determined parameters. All of the networks appeared to have approximately the correct number of weights since in the first (GLM) network the number of well-determined parameters was 9.0, or 90%, of ten weights (one each from the nine predictors plus the bias); the second (hidden layer) network had 60.3 well-determined parameters (90%) of the 67 weights; the transforming had 73.8 well-determined parameters (90%) of 82 weights. If the number of well-determined parameters is much less than the number of weights it suggests that the network design should be simplified.

There was very little to choose between the networks, with respect to training times, so the only criterion on which they can be compared and judged is their ability to correctly classify cases, plus any benefit that they may offer over a GLM. Accuracy was assessed, separately, for both the training and testing data using four criteria: the numbers of false positive (benign cases misidentified as malignant) and negative (malignant cases misidentified as benign) cases; Nagelkerke's R^2; and what NevProp calls a c-index. The c-index is related to the area under a ROC curve (AUC, Section 7.7). A value of 1 indicates that classes are separated perfectly while a value of 0.5 indicates that the classifier is performing no better than guessing. The results are given in Table 6.3. The 'rules' by which the network identified the two classes were investigated using NevProp's ARD (automatic relevance detection) statistics and the raw input-hidden and hidden-output weights that Olden *et al.* (2004) identified as the best methodology for quantifying variable importance. These results, plus some information from the earlier logistic regression analysis, are given in Table 6.4.

Table 6.3. *Accuracy statistics for three neural networks ('glm', 'hidden' and 'transform')
predicting the cancer class from nine predictors. Statistics are given for the training
and testing data*

Network	False-positives		False-negatives		c-index		Nagelkerke's R^2	
	training	testing	training	testing	training	testing	training	testing
glm	8	6	8	2	0.996	0.997	0.934	0.934
hidden	7	2	7	2	0.996	0.997	0.951	0.930
transform	7	3	8	2	0.994	0.997	0.945	0.924

Table 6.4. *Variable importance measures for three neural networks ('glm', 'hidden' and
'transform') and a logistic regression (Section 5.4.3)*

Predictor	Connection weights			ARD statistics			Logistic regression		
	glm	hidden	transform	glm	hidden	transform	z value	Exp(b)	Coefficient (b)
Clump thickness	−0.593	−2.456	−2.089	30.29	25.00	16.82	3.767	1.707	0.535
Uniformity of cell size	0.052	−0.924	−1.017	0.27	4.04	12.64	−0.03	0.994	−0.006
Uniformity of cell shape	−0.148	−1.147	−1.190	1.98	5.77	14.01	1.399	1.381	0.323
Marginal adhesion	−0.270	−1.093	−0.412	6.28	5.11	3.96	2.678	1.392	0.331
Single epithelial cell size	0.015	−0.318	−0.325	0.01	0.26	2.57	0.617	1.101	0.097
Bare nuclei	−0.457	−2.221	−2.033	29.03	32.87	24.43	4.082	1.467	0.383
Bland chromatin	−0.415	−1.723	−1.737	10.34	8.76	14.96	2.609	1.564	0.447
Nucleoli	−0.311	−1.339	−0.969	9.48	8.43	10.43	1.887	1.237	0.213
Mitoses	−0.635	−2.564	−0.027	12.31	9.76	0.17	1.627	1.707	0.535

Table 6.3 shows that there is very little to choose between the three neural networks, with respect to accuracy. Encouragingly, the performance with the test data was as good, or better, than the training data. This suggests that the networks are not over-trained. There is some suggestion that including transformations helps to improve the test-set accuracy, but the improvements could only ever be marginal given the accuracy of the 'glm' network. On the evidence from these analyses there is little to be gained from using a neural

network with these data. If the variable importance measures are compared (Table 6.4) there is considerable agreement between the two neural network measures and the logistic regression coefficients, albeit with opposite signs. Indeed the correlation between the connection weights and the logistic regression coefficients is −0.932. With the exception of the transforming neural network and the GAM (Section 5.6), mitoses was one of the three most important predictors. In the transforming neural network and the GAM, mitoses was the least important predictor. Clump thickness was either the first or second most important predictor across all analyses except for the GAM where it was the fifth. This was also one of the four predictors selected by the decision tree (Section 6.2.2). Uniformity of cell size and shape were consistently ranked towards the bottom of the list of importance. This is an interesting comparison to the decision tree in which uniformity of cell size was the first predictor used and uniformity of cell shape was one of the four selected.

The fact that the hidden and transforming networks only had marginal impacts on the accuracy of the predictors suggests that there is little need to consider including either transformations or interactions in the logistic regression. The correlation between the logistic regression coefficients and the connection weights in the 'hidden' network is also large (0.852), again suggesting that little was gained from the extra versatility provided by the hidden layer. There is less agreement between the 'glm' or 'hidden' ARD statistics and the logistic regression coefficients, perhaps supporting the view of Olden *et al.* (2004) that the connection weight measure is the best summary of the relative importance of the variables. The most significant change in importance, when the transforming layer was used, relates to the mitoses predictor. Neither the GAM, nor the decision tree, identified this as an important predictor yet it was the first or second most important in the linear analyses.

These analyses followed the outline suggested by Goodman and Harrell (2001a,b) and the general conclusion is that a standard generalised linear regression is sufficient, although it may be worth exploring a transformation for the mitoses predictor. They also illustrate the important fact that neural networks are not necessarily black-box predictors and that there are methods available that appear to provide reliable evidence for the relative importance of the predictors.

6.4.7   Self-organising maps
Outline

The Self-organising map (SOM) algorithm was developed by Kohonen (1988, 1990) during the 1980s as an approach to the problem of automated speech recognition. It is an unsupervised learning method and is therefore similar to the methods described in Chapter 3. However, the algorithm is generally considered to be an artificial neural network, although it can also be viewed as a general iterative approach. One of the important differences from most unsupervised clustering methods is that it represents the clusters on a grid, with similar clusters in close proximity to each other. In some respects it is intermediate between hierarchical and k-means approaches because the number of clusters is not fixed in advance but it is constrained not to exceed the number of cells in the grid. SOM networks are being quite widely used in the interpretation of gene expression profiles.

A SOM can be viewed as two-layered network, with the first being an input layer consisting of one node per variable. Each node in the input layer is connected to every node in the second, Kohonen, layer. The size, and shape, of this layer is set by the analyst and will be a rectangular or hexagonal grid. The input nodes connect to the Kohonen layer via weights that are adjusted during the training phase. The values from each case are known as input vectors and, because each input node is connected to each Kohonen node, the input vectors are delivered in parallel to the second layer. The algorithm calculates how far, as a Euclidean distance, each Kohonen node's weights are from the input vector. The node with the smallest distance, i.e. its weights are the closest match to the input vector, is identified as the winner in a competitive learning situation and its weights are updated to increase the chance that the winning node will win again given the same input vector. An important difference from other neural network algorithms is that the weights of the winner's neighbours are also updated. The shape of the neighbourhood is determined by the analyst but is usually Gaussian. The weights are updated according to a rule that incorporates the distance from the winning node. In other words the adjustment will tend to be larger when distances are small. The actual adjustment also depends on the current magnitude of the learning rate. The learning rate at the beginning of the training is large to allow for coarse modifications to the network. However, the learning rate gradually decreases during the training phase to ensure that the network stabilises and maps local patterns. The size of the update region, i.e. the identity of the updated neighbouring nodes, is also important because if it is too large small clusters may not be found and if it is too small large-scale patterns may not be captured. As with the learning rate the solution is to begin with a large update region which is gradually reduced during training.

Although the SOM algorithm does not suffer from the same problems as the hierarchical clustering algorithms there are still problems with identifying class boundaries. It would be unwise to treat each grid in the Kohonen layer as a separate cluster. Almost certainly clusters will be spread across several adjacent nodes. The difficulty is deciding which nodes should be grouped together to form clusters. The mechanisms that have been suggested to identify the class boundaries all involve some post-processing of the clustering results.

Example analysis

This example uses the *som* function (version 0.3−4) from the R package to analyse Fisher's *Iris* data (Section 2.10). The commands used to produce the analysis are outlined below. The data file is available from the R dataset library. The fifth column of the *Iris* data set contains the species names which can be removed by creating a subset of the original data set.

```
iris.data <- iris[-c(5)]
```

The four predictors are next normalized to have a mean of zero and a standard deviation of one.

```
iris.data.n <- normalize(iris.data, byrow=F)
```

The SOM is now completed using a four by three grid with a rectangular topology and a Gaussian neighbourhood.

```
iris.som <- som(iris.data.n, xdim = 4, ydim =3, topol="rect",
neigh="gaussian")
```

The results are summarised by a plot (plot(iris.som)) which shows how the cases are spread between the 12 nodes in the Kohonen layer. More detailed information about individual cases and the network structure, which are not shown here, can be obtained using the print command (print(iris.som)). Figure 6.12 is an edited version of the plot produced by R.

Nodes one, five and nine contain the 50 *I. setosa* cases which are, as in all other analyses, separated from the other two species which overlap in the right-hand clusters. Nodes two, six and ten are empty.

6.5   Genetic algorithms

6.5.1   *Introduction*

Suppose that we have a difficult problem and we do not know how to begin finding a reasonable solution. One unlikely approach would be to begin with a collection (population) of random solutions. As long as the performance of each of these solutions (their fitness) can be measured it is possible to rank them. If these candidate solutions could be coded as a series of discrete entities (genes) then 'better' solutions may be found by breeding a next generation of solutions.

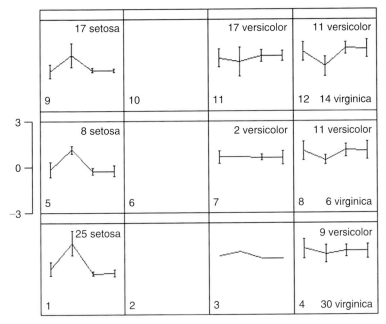

Figure 6.12 Plot of the distribution of cases across the Kohonen network. Nodes are numbered from the lower left. The *y*-axis scale has standard normal deviate units and shows the mean values for the four variables: sepal length and width and petal length and width. (Additional information on the number of cases from each species has been added to the plot.)

Hopefully, some of these offspring will produce even better solutions. If this is continued long enough a large space of potential solutions will have been searched which could lead to the identification of an optimal solution. If some biologically inspired processes, such as cross-overs and mutations, are included this will introduce the necessary variability to the solutions, whilst simultaneously avoiding becoming stuck at local maxima. This approach to developing classifiers is known as a genetic algorithm (GA).

There are some important terms that reflect their biologically inspired background. As in biology the population is a group of individuals (classifiers in these examples) that have the potential to exchange genetic information through mating. The most accurate classifiers produce the most offspring for the next generation. Each classifier, or individual, has a *fitness* level, which would be the accuracy of its predictions. The difficult part of a genetic algorithm is coding the classifier's structure as a set of 'genes'. Depending on the implementation the genes may be binary bit-strings or an array of numbers. Each gene represents a discrete part of the classifier which could be, for example, the value of a coefficient or logical operator. The system is allowed to evolve over a large number of discrete generations; in reality this is an iterative algorithm with each generation being one iteration. The population is evaluated at the end of each generation and the next generation of candidate solutions is formed from offspring that are based on that evaluation. The important difference between a GA and other iterative search algorithms is that the structure of the classifier is allowed to change during mating. Normally iterative search algorithms adjust the values of parameters by a direction and amount that is determined by the current lack of fit. The changes in the individual classifiers, within a GA, are not constrained in a similar way. Indeed some changes will produce offspring classifiers that have much lower accuracy than their parents.

Classifiers are modified via the usual genetic recombination operators: mutation and crossover. Mutations are random changes to the value of a gene. For example, a coefficient could increase in size while an arithmetic operator could switch from addition to subtraction. The crossover operator swaps information between classifiers. This could mean, for example, that an offspring classification rule would contain the left part of one parent's classifier function combined with the right part of the other parent's classifier. Because the classifiers are graded during each generation, and the better ones have an increased probability of producing offspring, it is expected that, over time, one or more good classifiers will evolve. However, one of the biggest difficulties with most GA implementations is finding a suitable way of coding the classifier as a series of discrete 'genes'. Although they are a little dated, the genetic algorithm FAQs (AI Repository, 1997) are still a good source of background information.

6.5.2   Genetic algorithms as classifiers

Stockwell (1992, 1993, 1999), Stockwell and Noble (1992) and Stockwell and Peters (1999) were some of the first to use GA as biological classifiers. The GARP (genetic algorithm for rule-set production) method (Stockwell and Noble, 1992) produces a variety of rule types to predict the distribution of a species. GARP has now evolved and is available for species distribution modelling from http://www.lifemapper.org/desktopgarp/, while Stockwell has expanded his ideas into his ambitious WhyWhere species mapping program (http://biodi.sdsc.edu/ww_home.html).

BEAGLE (biological evolutionary algorithm generating logical expressions) is an early genetic algorithm developed by Forsyth (1981) that has been used several times as a classifier in a biological context. For example, Fox et al. (1994) used BEAGLE to generate a set of rules that could be used to predict the presence/absence of pochard Aythya ferina on gravel pit lakes in southern Britain.

Fielding and Haworth (1995) investigated the generality of predictive models (logistic regression and discriminant analysis) for predicting the distribution of golden eagle *Aquila chrysaetos* nest sites. They identified several problems, including a lack of generality and a failure to achieve reciprocal accuracy between different regions of Scotland. One of their suggestions was that other machine learning methods may be more capable of achieving the desired generality. Fielding (1999a) used BEAGLE to generate rules for a rule-based expert system (Filho *et al.*, 1994) that could be used to predict the presence of eagle nests from the same data set. The following four rules that BEAGLE identified did have better cross-region predictive accuracy.

```
1.  (Calluna AND ((Rugged terrain > 5.8) OR (Wet heath >= 5.0)))
2.  ((Improved  grassland  <>  semi-improved  grassland)<(((Post
    canopy forest - Steep terrain) > 6.9 > Post canopy forest))
3.  (((Rocky outcrops = 0) OR (Bog <= 2.0)) < (Land below 200m <= 12.5))
4.  (Flat terrain < 7.1) AND (Pre-canopy forest + Sea) < 7.9))
```

It seems that some of this increased generality resulted from the incorporation of OR operators into the rules which makes allowances for regional differences in habitat availability and choice. It is also possible to rank the classifiers in terms of their ease of interpretation. It is usually relatively simple to translate statistical models into ecological models; neural network models are more difficult. In some cases the BEAGLE rules can be converted to simple ecological relationships, for example the first golden eagle rule, others are more obscure.

Jeffers (1996, 1999) describes the use of BEAGLE and GAFFER (South, 1994) as classifiers. GAFFER (genetic algorithm for finding existing relationships) is similar to BEAGLE in that it generates rule sets; however, unlike BEAGLE, it can be applied directly to multi-class and regression-type problems. Jeffers (1996) describes BEAGLE as an alternative to statistical methods for predicting the class of leaves from the elm genus. Jeffers (1999) extends the examples and includes an illustration of using GAFFER to predict the species of *Iris* from the floral measurements (Section 2.10). As shown in the previous analyses it is easy to separate *I. setosa* from the other two species and both BEAGLE and GAFFER identified one rule: petal length < sepal width. If this rule is true the species is *I. setosa*. BEAGLE can only be used for binary splits and it found two rules that were successful at separating *I. versicolor* from *I. virginica*. The first rule ((petal length − sepal width) < 1.64) or ((petal length + petal width) < 7.36), has a 98% success rate across the whole data set while the second rule (petal width < 1.62) and (petal length < 4.96), has an overall accuracy of 97%.

There are several points to note from these rules that were also apparent in the earlier golden eagle rules. Firstly, they incorporate logical operators. They also combine variables in a variety of ways. Finally, they use thresholds, which mean that a rule has preconditions that determine when it can be applied. If these conditions are not met, the rule is not used. This is similar to a decision tree but represents an important difference from the usual general linear model. Finally, the fact that two very different rules, with almost equal accuracy, were produced emphasises that there are often several possible classifiers with almost the same accuracy, but different interpretations.

Jeffer's (1999) use of GAFFER with the *Iris* data reinforced the point about alternative classifiers. Because GAFFER can discriminate between multiple classes it produced alternative rule sets that included all three species. The first rule, which has very simple conditions had an error rate of about 5%.

```
If (petal length < sepal width) then Iris setosa
else, if (petal length < 4.81) then Iris versicolor
else, Iris virginica.
```

Two other rule sets had similar accuracy but the second one is more complex.

```
If (petal length => sepal width) then
  if (petal width => 1.65) Iris virginica
  else, Iris versicolor
else, Iris setosa.
If (petal length => sepal width), then
  if (petal width > sqrt(sepal width)) Iris virginica
  else, Iris versicolor
  else, Iris setosa.
```

Jeffers (1999) commented on these alternative rule sets by noting that users were often disconcerted by the ability of the algorithms to find more than one rule set which had a similar accuracy. However, he suggested that this is an advantage of a rule-based approach which conforms to the logic of the scientific method and affirms that there may well be many possible hypotheses between which we are unable to distinguish with the available data. He also warns that it is a salutatory lesson that many users of statistical methods should bear in mind when interpreting their statistical models, which will be constrained by their algorithm to always find the same rule given a set of data. Li *et al.* (2003) made use of a similar property of multiple rule sets for cancer diagnosis. However, their rules were not derived from a genetic algorithm, instead they used multiple instances of a decision tree that used differently ranked predictors in the root node.

6.5.3   Feature selection using a GA

Although algorithms such as BEAGLE and GARP have been used to generate classifiers, one of the most common roles for GA is in classifier refinement, for example setting parameters such as the size of the hidden layer in a neural network and selecting the 'best' predictors to be used with the final classifier. Inevitably this creates a significant computational load, but this is likely to become less significant as computing power continues to increase. It is also important to recognise the balance between the resources, including time, needed to collect the data and the resources needed to analyse them. An extra few days analysing data that took months to collect, should not be viewed as a major disadvantage.

Four examples that attempt to optimise the selection of genes as predictors in cancer classifications are listed below. Liu *et al.* (2005) used a GA to select genes for a SVM that was used in a cancer multi-class recognition problem. Using this feature selection procedure reduced the number of predictor genes from 16 063 to 40 and yet still allowed accurate multi-class tumour identifications. However, they also note that the random nature of the GA resulted in the production of different independent sets of predictive genes. The existence of multiple sets of predictor genes is analogous to the multiple rule sets reported by Jeffers (1999), and it raises questions about their explanatory value even though they have predictive power. Jirapech-Umpai and Aitken (2005) used a GA to select sets of genes for a k-NN classifier. They used two approaches: the first allowed genes to be added or deleted while the second changed the weighting for individual genes between zero (do not use) and one (use). Deb and Reddy (2003), in a detailed description of their approach, used a GA to optimise the predictors for the classification of two classes of cancer. Their GA simultaneously optimised three objectives: minimising the number of predictors; minimising the number of incorrectly classified cases in the training data; and minimising the number of misclassified cases in the test data. Karzynski *et al.* (2003) combined a GA with a SOM to obtain a reduced number of gene expression values for their classifier and highlighted the superiority of the GA approach for predictor selection because of its ability to select genes that were individually bad predictors but which become good predictors when combined with others.

6.6   Others

6.6.1   Case-based reasoning

Case-based reasoning (CBR) is a methodology that is often linked with expert systems and aims to model human reasoning and thinking. Two of its biggest advantages are said to be its ability to improve with time, as more cases are added, and its ability to adapt to changes in its data environment. CBR algorithms are based around the principle of recognising similarities with problems or cases that have been solved or identified in the past. This is achieved by matching possible 'solutions' to a database of earlier examples. If a match or partial match is found an answer can be provided; alternatively the database can be adapted (revised) to take account of 'new' information. One very important part of a CBR algorithm is the measurement of similarity. This is usually achieved by calculating a bounded similarity measure that has a range from zero (very different) to one (very similar). Because there is no constraint on datatypes these similarities do not necessarily make use of quantitative concepts such as Euclidean distances. In addition, account must be taken of the relative 'importance' of each variable. This is achieved by calculating an overall similarity measure that is a weighted average of all of the individual similarities. Watson and Marir (1994) is a comprehensive, although rather old, review of CBR methods and applications from the ai-cbr website. The ai-cbr site is no longer updated but does still contain some useful resources for CBR methods.

Although CBR has been shown to be successful in commercial applications there do not appear to be many biological applications. However, Remm (2004) showed how CBR could be used for species and habitat mapping while Armengol and Plaza (2003) described a new similarity measure and tested it with an application to assess the carcinogenic activity of chemicals from a toxicology database.

6.6.2   Nearest neighbour

These are conceptually simple, and one of the oldest, classifiers. They belong to a class of instance-based learning methods which differ from other classification methods because they do not build a classifier until a new unknown case needs to be classified. The class of a case is the majority class (vote) of its nearest neighbours. However, this definition raises three questions. Firstly, how is distance measured to find the nearest neighbours; secondly, how many neighbours should be examined; and finally, are all neighbours equal? Surprisingly, using only one neighbour appears to be quite successful. If many neighbours are used the number of neighbours in each class is a measure of the local class posterior probabilities.

One objective method of determining the number of neighbours (k) is by cross-validation. A range of values for k is used and each case is classified by the majority vote of its k nearest neighbours. The classification accuracy is checked and the best k value is the one with the lowest cross-validated accuracy.

The distance function, and the predictors, will have a large effect on the classifier's performance. As with many classifiers, the inclusion of uninformative predictors (noise) can degrade its performance which means that predictor selection algorithms, along with all of their problems, must be employed.

Neighbours do not need to make the same contribution to the final vote. Unequal class proportions create difficulties because the majority vote rule will tend to favour the larger class. One way of dealing with this is to weight neighbours by their class prior probabilities. Voting contributions can also be adjusted according to misclassification costs. Finally, it seems reasonable to weight the votes by their nearness. Close neighbours have a larger weight than more distant ones.

As with all of the other classifiers described there are many extensions including some that combine the nearest neighbour classifier with decision trees. Hall and Samworth (2005) demonstrated that their performance (accuracy) could be improved by bagging (Section 4.7). However, the resample size had to be less than 69% of the original sample if the resampling used a with-replacement method, and less than 50% for without-replacement.

Yeang *et al.* (2001) is an example where a k-NN method was used, in conjunction with others, to investigate the potential for classifying multiple tumour types from molecular data and Jirapech-Umpai and Aitken (2005) used a GA to select sets of genes for their k-NN classifier which predicted the class from microarray data.

6.6.3   Combined classifiers

Different classifiers can have quite different characteristics. This means that, for a given set of training data, their predictions may not match. This is not necessarily a problem since it enables their predictions to be combined which may produce a better overall performance. Although there are other techniques, the main method of combining classifiers runs them in parallel and then passes their predictions on to a 'combiner'. A combiner is an algorithm which pools together the predictions to arrive at a consensus classification for each case. The simplest combiner uses votes to determine the prediction, while other more complex algorithms may weight a classifier's predictions depending on the composition of the training data (training data may vary if they were derived using resampling or boosting methods).

6.7   Where next?

In view of the differences between the classifiers described in this and the previous chapter it is reasonable to ask which is the best and are some more appropriate for particular types of problem than others. Although it is difficult to compare classifiers (see Section 7.9), comparative studies rarely find major performance benefits, at least as measured by their overall accuracy. This means that other criteria have to be used to decide between them. An ideal classifier (Fielding, 2002) would be accurate, with utility and an ability to handle costs (Section 7.8). Since most classifiers have approximately the same accuracy and can incorporate costs, either implicitly or explicitly, the choice appears to rest with their utility.

Two important utility criteria are scalability and transparency. Scalability is measured by the performance degradation, as measured in the time taken to arrive at an answer, as the dataset increases in size. Generally, performance will only be an important criterion when real-time class identification is required. The second measure, transparency, relates to the acceptance of the findings by one's peers. There is some evidence, at least within ecology (Fielding, unpublished results), that the choice of a classifier is affected by the author's location, the habitat and the taxonomic group. For example, artificial neural networks appear to be widely used in freshwater biology studies and not very often in avian ecology, while decision trees appear most often in papers authored by people working in North America. This suggests that the selection of a classifier may not be based on objective criteria, rather it reflects what is acceptable by workers in that area. There is sometimes a tendency to equate scientific acceptability with complexity. I particularly like this quote from H. J. S. Smith: 'It is the peculiar beauty of this method gentlemen, and one which endears it to the really scientific mind, that under no circumstances can it be of the smallest possible utility.' Although this almost certainly overstates the case, it has a germ of truth. If a classifier, and its predictions, is to be accepted by an informed, but non-specialist, audience transparency is essential. Three of the methods (artificial neural networks, SVM and genetic algorithms) described in this chapter are likely to fail this test while decision trees and CBR have simple relationships that are easy to understand. However, most of the methods, including decision trees and CBR, require many design decisions that often go undocumented and unjustified. These design decisions have significant impacts on the classifier's performance and their subsequent generality (see Chapter 7). However, the design decisions may not be independent of the designer's preconceptions about the problem leading to a potential invisible bias. Section 7.9 discusses the various approaches that have been used to compare classifiers.

7

Classification accuracy

7.1 Background

Probably the most important aim for any classifier is that it should make accurate predictions. However, it is surprisingly difficult to arrive at an adequate definition and measurement of accuracy (see Fielding and Bell, 1997; Fielding, 1999b, 2002). Also, it may be better to think in terms of costs rather than accuracy and use a minimum cost criterion to evaluate the effectiveness of a classifier. Unfortunately costs have rarely been used (explicitly) in biological studies and it is reasonable to expect some opposition to their future use. However, in Section 7.8 it is shown that all classifiers apply costs that may have gone unrecognised.

Ultimately the only test of any classifier is its future performance, i.e. its ability to classify correctly novel cases. This is known as generalisation and it is linked to both classifier design and testing. In general, complex classifiers are fine tuned to re-classify the cases used in developmental testing. As such they are likely to incorporate too much of the 'noise' from the original cases, leading to a decline in accuracy when presented with novel cases. It is sometimes necessary to accept reduced accuracy on the training data if it leads to increased accuracy with novel cases. This was illustrated in the decision tree and artificial neural network sections in Chapter 6. Focusing on the generalisation of a classifier differs from traditional statistical approaches which are usually judged by the coefficient p-values or some overall goodness of fit such as R^2. The statistical focus relates to the goodness of fit of the data to some pre-defined model and does not explicitly test performance on future data, generally because of the assumptions made about the parameters estimated by the statistics. Instead it may be better to follow Altman and Royston's (2000) suggestion that 'Usefulness is determined by how well a model works in practice, not by how many zeros there are in the associated P-values'.

7.2   Appropriate metrics

Accuracy is measured by some metric, the most obvious being the percentage of cases correctly classified (CCR). However, imagine that one wants to develop a classifier that can detect abnormal cells in a tissue sample. These abnormal cells are present in approximately 1% of the population. It is possible to get an impressive percentage correct with very little effort. Indeed, the classifier's performance will get even better as the percentage of affected people declines. The trivial classification rule is that all samples are normal, giving 99% accuracy with a 1% abnormality prevalence. If the prevalence is 1 in 1000 the rule has an even better 99.9% accuracy. The rule is, of course, useless. The classifier is very accurate but has no utility. However, it is difficult to imagine a useful classifier that could approach this level of accuracy. As long as the prevalence is below 0.5 a CCR of $>50\%$ is guaranteed by the simple majority rule.

Imagine another pair of classifiers that do not use trivial rules. The aim of these classifiers is to identify species as 'safe' or 'extinction prone'. The test data consist of 100 species which are evenly split between the two classes, i.e. 50 'safe' and 50 'at risk'. This time a trivial rule would only be expected to get 50% of the predictions correct. Both classifiers are 75% accurate. Which is the best? Of course, this question cannot be answered without additional information. Classifier A got 40% of the 'at risk' predictions wrong while B got the same percentage of the 'safe' predictions wrong and 10% of the 'at risk' predictions wrong. Even though their overall performance was identical, most people would argue that B was better because it had fewer of the most costly mistakes. As in the previous example the two prediction errors do not carry the same cost.

These examples demonstrate that there is a context to predictions which must be included in any metric. The next section identifies some of the more common accuracy metrics and identifies some limitations.

7.3   Binary accuracy measures

The simplest classifiers make binary predictions (yes/no, malignant/ benign, present/absence, etc.). There are two possible prediction errors in a two-class problem: false positives and false negatives and the performance of a binary classifier is normally summarised in a confusion or error matrix (Figure 7.1) that cross-tabulates the observed and predicted presence/absence patterns as

Actual class

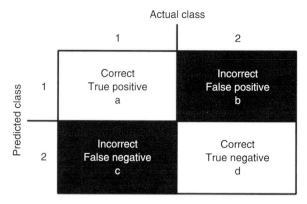

Figure 7.1 A generic confusion matrix.

four numbers: a, b, c and d. Although data in the confusion matrix are sometimes presented as percentages, all of the derived measures in Table 7.1 are based on counts.

The simplest measure of prediction accuracy from the confusion matrix is the proportion of cases that are classified correctly, the CCR: $(a + d)/(a + b + c + d)$. However, it is possible to derive many other measures from the four cell counts (Table 7.1).

The measures in Table 7.1 have different characteristics. For example, sensitivity, which measures the proportion of correctly classified positive cases, takes no account of the false positives. Conversely specificity measures the false positive errors (see Altman and Bland, 1994). The odds ratio, which is the ratio of presence to absence, has some interesting properties that make it useful in other situations (see Bland and Altman, 2000). However, it can be tricky to interpret.

Some of the measures in Table 7.1 are sensitive to the prevalence (p) of positive cases and some can be used to measure the improvement over chance. For example, with high prevalence it is possible to achieve a high CCR by the simple expedient of assigning all cases to the most common group. Kappa (K), which is the proportion of specific agreement, is often used to assess improvement over chance. Landis and Koch (1977) suggested that $K < 0.4$ indicates poor agreement, whilst a value above 0.4 is indicative of good agreement. However, K is sensitive to the sample size and it is unreliable if one class dominates. The tau coefficient (Ma and Redmond, 1995) is a related measure but it depends on a priori knowledge of the prevalence rather the a posteriori estimate used by K. Although the related NMI measure does not suffer from these problems it shows non-monotonic behaviour under conditions of excessive errors (Forbes, 1995).

Table 7.1. *Confusion matrix-derived accuracy measures.* N *is the number of cases* (a+b+c+d)

Measure	Calculation
Correct classification rate	$(a + d)/N$
Misclassification rate	$(b + c)/N$
Overall diagnostic power	$(b + d)/N$
Sensitivity	$a/(a + c)$
Positive predictive power	$a/(a + b)$
Specificity	$d/(b + d)$
Negative predictive power	$d/(c + d)$
False-positive rate	$b/(b + d)$
False-negative rate	$c/(a + c)$
Odds ratio	$(ad)/(cb)$
Kappa statistic	$\dfrac{(a + d) - \{[(a + c)(a + b) + (b + d)(c + d)]/N\}}{N - \{[(a + c)(a + b) + (b + d)(c + d)]/N\}}$
NMI	$1 - \dfrac{\left\{ \begin{array}{c} a.\ln(a) - b.\ln(b) - c.\ln(c) - d.\ln(d) \\ +(a + b).\ln(a + b) + (c + d).\ln(c + d) \end{array} \right\}}{N.\ln N - [(a + c).\ln(a + c) + (b + d).\ln(b + d)]}$

It is also important to use measures that quantify agreement and not association. For example, a classifier that got all cases wrong would show perfect association but no agreement. Calculating a chi-squared statistic for the following two confusion matrices yields the same value (chi-squared $= 162$) even though the relationships are inverted:

$$
\begin{array}{cc} 5 & 95 \\ 95 & 5 \end{array} \qquad \begin{array}{cc} 95 & 5 \\ 5 & 95 \end{array}
$$

Huberty (1994, p. 105) described a one-tailed test that can be used to test if a classifier's performance is better than could be obtained by chance by determining if the observed (O) and expected (E) correct classification rates differ significantly:

$$O = a + d$$
$$E = p(a + c) + (1 - p)(b + d)$$

where p is the prevalence of positive cases. From these values a z score can be obtained from $z = (O - E) \sqrt{(E(N - E)/N)}$. If p is low the calculation of E can be adjusted to $(1 - p)N$. This enables a test of improvement over the rate achieved using the trivial rule of assigning all cases to the negative group.

7.4   Appropriate testing data

Although there are legitimate concerns about which of the previous measures should be used to assess the predictive accuracy of a classifier there are even greater concerns about which data should be used for its calculation. A classifier has little merit if its predictions cannot be, or are not, assessed for their accuracy using independent data. In other words it is important to have some idea about how well the classifier will perform with new data. This is important because the accuracy achieved with the original data is often much greater than that achieved with new data (Henery, 1994). Consequently, it is generally accepted that robust measures of a classifier's accuracy must make use of independent data, i.e. data not used to develop the classifier. The two data sets needed to develop and test predictions are known by a variety of synonyms. The terms 'training' and 'testing' data are used here. The problem now becomes one of finding appropriate training and testing data. A more robust test uses three data sets: training, validation and testing. The training and validation sets are equivalent to the training and testing sets in the two-set example. When there are three data sets the test set is not used until the final classifier has been developed. In this way it is not used to tune the performance of the classifier and therefore provides a more independent test of performance.

7.4.1   Re-substitution

The simplest, and least satisfactory, way of testing the performance of a classifier is to apply it to the data that were used to develop it. This method is called re-substitution. The problem is that re-substitution provides a biased over-assessment of the classifier's future performance. One explanation for this is that the form of the classifier may have been determined by some model-selection method (equivalent to stepwise selection of predictor variables in a multiple regression). An inevitable consequence of the model selection process is that the final model tends to 'over-fit' the training data because the classifier has been optimised to deal with the nuances in the training data. This bias may still apply if the same set of 'independent' testing data has been used to verify the model selection (Chatfield, 1995). Lin and Pourhmadi (1998) suggested that extensive 'data mining' for the appropriate model produces small prediction errors for the training data but at the cost of a significant loss of generality. Consequently, the best assessment of a classifier's future value is to test it with some truly independent data; ideally a sample that was collected independently of the training data (this is usually termed 'prospective sampling'). However, a common practice in machine learning studies is to apply some technique that splits or partitions the available data to provide the training and the 'independent' testing data. Unfortunately, arbitrarily partitioning the existing data is not as effective as collecting new data.

7.4.2   Hold-out

At its simplest, partitioning involves the splitting of data into two unequally sized groups. The largest partition is used for training while the second, or hold-out, sample is used for testing. In reality, this type of data splitting is just a special case of a broader class of more computationally intensive approaches that split the data into two or more groups.

Huberty (1994) provided a rule of thumb for determining the ratio of training to testing cases that is based on the work of Schaafsma and van Vark (1979). This heuristic, which is restricted to presence/absence models, suggests a ratio of $[1 + (p - 1)^{1/2}]^{-1}$, where p is the number of predictors. For example, if $p = 10$ the testing set should be $1/[1 + \sqrt{9}]$, or 0.25, of the complete data set. An increase in the number of predictors is matched by an increase in the proportion of cases needed for training, thus if there are 17 predictors 80% of cases are required for training.

7.4.3   Cross-validation

When the performance of a classifier is assessed we do not obtain its actual error rate, rather it is estimated from an apparent confusion matrix that was obtained, ideally, from a randomly selected member of the possible testing set(s) (Blayo *et al.*, 1995). Both the re-substitution and hold-out methods suffer because they are single estimates of the classifier's accuracy with no indication of its precision. Estimates of precision are only possible when there is more than one data point. However, because the number of available test sets is frequently small the error rate estimates are likely to be imprecise with wide confidence intervals. It can also be shown that a classifier which uses all of the available data will, on average, perform better than a classifier based on a subset. Consequently, because partitioning inevitably reduces the size of training set there will usually be a corresponding decrease in the classifier's accuracy. Conversely larger test sets reduce the variance of the error estimates if more than one test set is available. There is, therefore, a trade-off between having large test sets that give a good assessment of the classifier's performance and small training sets which are likely to result in a poor classifier. Rencher (1995) suggested that while partitioning should be used for model validation, all available data should be used to develop the eventual classification rule. These guidelines relate to the need to develop a classifier that has low bias and low variance.

One way of obtaining multiple test sets is to split the available data into three or more partitions. The first of these methods, *k*-fold partitioning, splits the data into k equal-sized partitions or folds. One fold is used as a test set whilst the remainder form the training set. This is repeated so that each fold forms a separate test set, yielding k measures of performance. The overall performance is then based on an average over these k test sets. The extreme value for k is obtained using the leave-one-out (L-O-O), and the related jack-knife, procedure. These give the best compromise between maximising the size of the training data set and providing a robust test of the classifier. In both methods each case is used sequentially as a single test sample, while the remaining $n-1$ cases form the training set. However, the L-O-O method can produce unreliable estimates because of the large variance.

Kohavi (1995) investigated the performance of various partitioning methods with six data sets and showed that k-fold partitioning was pessimistically biased for low values of k, but when $k = 10$ the estimates were reasonable and almost unbiased for $k = 20$. His recommendation, based on a method which combined reasonable values for the bias and variance, was that 10-fold partitioning produced the best results, as long as the folds were stratified. The folds are stratified when the class proportions are approximately the same as those in the complete data set. This approach works because stratifying the folds tends to reduce the variance of the estimates.

7.4.4   *Bootstrapping methods*

The hold-out and L-O-O methods are two extremes of a continuum which have different variance and bias problems. One way of overcoming these problems is to replace both with a large number of bootstrapped samples (random sampling with replacement; Efron and Tibshirani, 1997). In this approach the classifier is run many times using a large number of training samples that are drawn at random, with replacement, from the single real training set. Because replacement sampling is used it is normal to have some cases represented several times in a bootstrap sample, while others are not used. It is possible to show that the probability that an individual case will not be included as a training example is $(1-1/n)^n$, where n is the number of bootstrapped training samples. Because $(1-1/n)^n$ is approximately equal to e^{-1} (0.368), it can also be shown that a particular case should be included in training cases $0.632n$ times. Using this information a less biased estimate can be found from $0.368e_b + 0.632e_x$, where e_b is the error from the training sets and e_x is the error for cases not included in the training set. While Jain *et al.* (1987) and others have demonstrated, experimentally, that bootstrap sampling is better than other cross-validation methods, Kohavi (1995) cautions that its low variance could be combined with a large bias for some, but not all, datasets. Wehrens *et al.* (2000) have a detailed description of bootstrapped error rates.

7.4.5   *Out-of-bag estimates*

Bootstrap aggregation, or bagging, are bootstrapping methods that give reasonable and unbiased accuracy estimates, particularly for unstable classifiers such as decision trees. Bootstrapped samples are generated such that a 'reasonable' proportion of cases are withheld from the training data. Typically about a third of the cases are withheld. Once the classifier has been built, using the bootstrapped sample data, it can be tested on the withheld fraction (the out-of-bag sample). If this is repeated many times each case will have a set of predictions from test samples. The final class prediction is the majority class for the out-of-bag predictions.

7.4.6   *Reject rates*

Jain *et al.* (2000) discuss a useful measure of classifier performance called the reject rate. This is the proportion of cases that the classifier's predictions fail to reach a 'certainty' threshold. If such a system is not applied some cases will be assigned to classes with very marginal probabilities of belonging to the class. There are many circumstances in which failure to reach a conclusion is better than a weakly supported conclusion. A general consequence of employing a reject rule is that overall accuracy, for the retained cases, increases.

7.5   **Decision thresholds**

Although many of the measures in Table 7.1 are much better than the simplistic CCR, they fail to make use of all of the available information. Often, the assignment of a case to a class depends on the application of a threshold to some score, for example the output from an artificial neuron. Inevitably this dichotomisation of the raw score results in the loss of information; in particular we do not know how marginal the assignments were. Thus, using a $0-1$ raw score scale and a 0.5 threshold, cases with scores of 0.499 and 0.001 would be assigned to the same group, while cases with scores of 0.499 and 0.501 would be placed in different groups. Consequently, if we are not going to work with the raw scores or some other continuous variable, there are several reasons why the threshold value should be examined. For example, because unequal group sizes can influence the scores for many of the classifier methods it may be necessary to adjust the threshold to compensate for this bias. Similarly, if false negative errors are more serious than false positive errors the threshold can be adjusted to decrease the false negative rate at the expense of an increased false positive error rate. Other thresholds could be justified that are dependent on the intended application of the classifier, for example a 'minimum acceptable error' or false negative criterion. However, adjusting the threshold (cut-point) does not have

Example   187

consistent effects on the measures in Table 7.1. For example, lowering the threshold increases sensitivity but decreases specificity. Consequently adjustments to the threshold must be made within the context for which the classifier is to be used. For example, in a conservation study, more false-positive predictions could be tolerated for a particularly endangered species, but if the role of the classifier was to identify sites where we could be certain of finding a species in a field survey, the threshold would need to be adjusted to minimise the false-positive error rates.

7.6   Example

The following example is used to illustrate most of the issues raised in the previous sections. The data are a subset of those used by Fielding and Haworth (1995). The aim was to construct a classifier (discriminant analysis) capable of predicting the location of golden eagle *Aquila chrysaetos* nest sites (current, alternative and historical (since 1960, $n = 60$) on the island of Mull. The results from a range of analyses are summarised in Table 7.2. Using these data there is very little difference between the results obtained using re-substitution (equal prior probabilities) and cross validation. Unfortunately we have to be cautious about both analyses because the large number of false positives has resulted in low PPP values. There is only a 12% chance that a predicted square actually contains a real nest. The kappa statistic is quite low, again suggesting that the classifier is not performing well. If the prior probabilities are changed to reflect the class sizes, i.e. 60/1117 and 1057/1117, the CCR rises to an impressive 94.4%. Unfortunately, the classifier can no longer correctly predict any real nest sites.

In the remainder of the analyses three partitioning schemes were used. The first applied Schaafsma and van Vark's (1979) rule, which uses the number of predictors to determine the proportion of cases needed for testing. Seventy-five percent of the cases were selected randomly for training. As might be expected the classifier performed better with the training data. The second scheme was a five-fold partitioning. No attempt was made to retain an equal number of nests within each partition. Although the mean values are quite similar to the previous results, it is interesting to note the range of values obtained for these five sets. When the second partition was used for testing the predictions were better than those obtained with the training data! When the fifth partition was used for testing there was a large discrepancy between the training and testing sensitivity values. These results illustrate clearly that the performance of a classifier is dependent on the composition of the training and testing sets.

The final partitioning scheme attempted to simulate prospective sampling. The island is split into three geographical regions that have quite distinct

Table 7.2. *Results obtained from various permutations of training and testing data sets for the Mull eagle data. (n = number of cases, tp = true positive, fn = false negative, fp = false positive, sensitivity = sensitivity (true positive fraction), PPP = positive predictive power, K = kappa, CCR = correct classification rate, EP = equal prior probabilities, CP = class size prior probabilities, cross-validated = leave-one-out testing. Approximately 75% of the data were selected randomly to form the training set, the remainder formed the test set; these proportions were determined using the rule suggested by Schaafsma and van Vark (1979).)*

	n	tp	fn	Sensitivity	fp	PPP	K	NMI	CCR (%)
Re-substitution[EP]	1117	44	16	0.73	317	0.12	0.13	0.10	70.2
Cross-validated	1117	42	18	0.70	320	0.12	0.12	0.08	69.7
Re-substitution[CP]	1117	0	60	0.00	3	0.00	0.00		94.4
75% training	855	33	11	0.75	244	0.12	0.13	0.10	70.2
25% testing	262	11	5	0.69	81	0.12	0.11	0.07	67.2
k-fold results, $k = 5$									
Train $k = 2, 3, 4, 5$	874	34	13	0.72	231	0.13	0.14	0.10	72.1
Test $k = 1$	243	9	4	0.69	79	0.10	0.09	0.06	65.8
Train $k = 1, 3, 4, 5$	895	33	16	0.67	246	0.12	0.12	0.08	70.7
Test $k = 2$	222	9	2	0.82	51	0.15	0.19	0.17	76.1
Train $k = 1, 2, 4, 5$	897	33	13	0.72	240	0.12	0.13	0.10	71.8
Test $k = 3$	220	8	6	0.57	45	0.15	0.15	0.07	76.8
Train $k = 1, 2, 3, 5$	892	36	13	0.73	255	0.12	0.13	0.10	70.0
Test $k = 4$	225	8	3	0.73	73	0.10	0.10	0.07	66.2
Train $k = 1, 2, 3, 4$	910	38	11	0.78	248	0.13	0.15	0.12	71.5
Test $k = 5$	207	6	5	0.54	63	0.09	0.06	0.03	67.1
Training data mean				0.72	244	0.12	0.13	0.10	71.2
Training data standard error				0.017	4.04	0.003	0.005	0.008	0.384
Testing data mean				0.67	14	0.12	0.12	0.08	70.4
Testing data standard error				0.050	6.410	0.014	0.022	0.025	2.480
Cross-region predictions									
Ben More	583	26	13	0.67	162	0.14	0.13	0.07	70.0
Test set	534	14	7	0.67	96	0.13	0.16	0.12	80.7
Ross of Mull	175	4	1	0.80	27	0.13	0.18	0.21	84.0
Test set	942	28	27	0.51	178	0.14	0.13	0.06	78.2
North Mull	359	11	5	0.69	68	0.14	0.17	0.13	79.7
Test set	758	41	3	0.93	312	0.12	0.12	0.14	58.4

Example   189

features arising from different geological conditions. The data from each region were used for training and the classifier was tested on the other two regions. These results illustrate some important points about accuracy assessment. For example, if the CCR is used as an index it is apparent that the North Mull classifier does not translate well to other regions. However, if sensitivity is used it is an excellent classifier. This discrepancy arises because almost half of the cases are labelled as false positives. Although it is not possible to illustrate this here (to protect the nest site locations) the false positives are clustered around the real nest sites. If a spatial correction is applied (Fielding and Bell, 1997) the CCR rises to 67%. When the Ross of Mull training data were used for training a high CCR, combined with good sensitivity, was obtained. However, the classifier performed poorly with the eagle nest site test data. Fielding and Haworth (1995) demonstrated that the cross-region predictive success for a range of raptors on the island of Mull, and the adjacent Argyllshire mainland, was dependent upon the particular combination of species, training and testing sets. There was no guarantee of reciprocity. Similar patterns of between-region predictive failure were also found for parrots on Wallacean islands (Marsden and Fielding, 1999).

In a final series of tests the effect of the allocation threshold was investigated. These tests used the classifier trained on 75% of the data. The results are summarised in Table 7.3. As expected changing the threshold alters the classification accuracy. Note that the value of the kappa statistic rises as the number of false positives declines. Unfortunately this is at the expense of true positives and is a consequence of the low prevalence of positive locations. Selecting the appropriate threshold for these data is dependent on the intended application.

Table 7.3. *Accuracy assessment after applying different thresholds to a discriminant score. tp = true positive, fn = false negative, fp = false positive, K = kappa (figures in italics have* $p > 0.05$*). See Table 7.2 for sample sizes. 0.46 is the default threshold.*

	Training, AUC = 0.798					Testing, AUC = 0.762				
Threshold	tp	fn	fp	K	PPP	tp	fn	fp	K	PPP
−0.92	44	0	662	0.023	0.06	15	1	200	*0.018*	0.07
−0.46	43	1	516	0.052	0.08	15	1	171	0.041	0.08
0.00	40	4	353	0.100	0.11	13	3	120	0.073	0.10
0.46	33	11	237	0.134	0.12	11	5	80	0.114	0.12
0.92	38	6	135	0.141	0.22	9	7	41	0.199	0.18
1.38	26	16	49	0.180	0.35	6	10	20	0.227	0.23
1.84	14	30	28	0.161	0.33	4	12	10	0.222	0.29

For example, to be reasonably certain of including 75% of nest sites in future samples the default threshold of 0.46 or below should be applied. Conversely, if resources were limited, the chances of finding a nest site in an unsurveyed area (large PPP) would be maximised by applying a threshold of 1.84 or above.

7.7   ROC plots

7.7.1   Background

An alternative solution to threshold adjustments is to make use of all the information contained within the original raw score and calculate measures that are threshold-independent. The receiver operating characteristic (ROC) plot is a threshold-independent measure that was developed as a signal-processing technique. The term refers to the performance (the operating characteristic) of a human or mechanical observer (the 'receiver') engaged in assigning cases into dichotomous classes (Deleo, 1993; Deleo and Campbell, 1990). ROC plots are described in the next section.

ROC plots have a long and extensive history in the analysis of medical diagnostic systems, as evidenced by Zou's (2002) comprehensive online bibliography. They have also been widely used, particularly recently, in machine learning studies. More recently, they have become one of the main methods used to assess the accuracy of ecological presence/absence models, following the recommendations by Fielding and Bell (1997). One of the main reasons for their adoption by these disciplines is their ability to deal with unequal class distributions and misclassification error costs. Fawcett (2003) has written an excellent guide to the use of ROC plots. Although it deals mainly with their use in comparing classifiers, it also provides a lot of useful practical and theoretical background.

A ROC plot shows the trade-offs between the ability to identify correctly true positives and the costs associated with misclassifying negative cases as positives (false positives). They have great versatility and can be used to investigate, for example:

- the effect of varying a decision threshold, i.e. the score used to split positive and negative cases;
- the variation in performance of a single classifier over a range of datasets;
- the relative performance of different classifiers on the same data set.

ROC plots have the great advantage of being insensitive to changes in prevalence. For example, if the proportion of positive cases changes the ROC plot

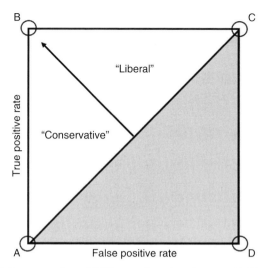

Figure 7.2 Interpretation of ROC space (based on Fawcett, 2003).

does not change. Fawcett's (2003) description of how the space within a ROC plot can be interpreted is summarised in Figure 7.2.

- The lower left point A (0, 0) is a classifier that never identifies any case as positive. While this would mean that there were no false-positive errors, all positive cases would be false-negative errors.
- The opposite corner, point C (1, 1), is the converse. All cases are labelled as positives and there are now no false-negative errors
- Point B (0, 1) is the ideal classifier with perfect classification.
- Point D (1, 0) would be a strange classifier which labelled every case incorrectly. Inverting the predictions would create a perfect classifier.
- The diagonal line running from A to C represents chance performance; the classifier would perform with the accuracy expected from tossing a coin. Any classifier in the grey area below this line is performing worse than chance.
- Any classifier whose performance in the upper left triangle is doing better than chance. Better classifiers are towards the point of the arrow.
- Classifiers that lie close to the A–C line can be tested to determine if their performance is significantly better than chance (see Forman, 2002).
- Classifiers to the left of the arrow are 'conservative', i.e. they make positive classifications only with strong evidence. While this means that there are few false-positive errors, they will also tend to misclassify many

of the positive cases as negative. This means that we can be reasonably certain about positive predictions but must be cautious with negative predictions.

- Classifiers to the right of the arrow are 'liberal', i.e. they make positive classifications with weak evidence. This means that they tend to get positive cases correct but at the expense of a high false-positive rate.

7.7.2   ROC curves

Not all classifiers provide the continuous values needed for a ROC plot. Consequently there is no opportunity to vary the thresholds and only a single confusion matrix is possible, producing a ROC plot with a single point (Figure 7.2). However, if raw scores are available they can be used to allocate cases to classes over a range of thresholds. This series of points, one per threshold, is then used to a produce a ROC curve.

A ROC curve is obtained by plotting all sensitivity values (true positive fraction), on the y axis, against their equivalent ($1 -$ specificity) values (false-positive fraction) for all available thresholds, on the x axis (Figure 7.3). The quality of the approximation to a curve depends on the number of thresholds tested. If a small number are tested the 'curve' will resemble a staircase. ROC curves should be convex but real ROC curves may have concave sections often resulting from small test sets.

The area under the ROC curve (AUC) is usually taken as the index of performance because it provides a single measure of overall accuracy that

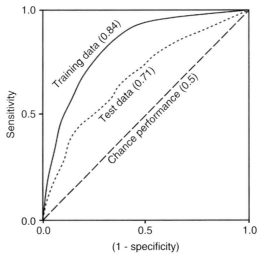

Figure 7.3 Example ROC curves (figures in parentheses are the AUC values).

is independent of any particular threshold (Deleo, 1993). The value of the AUC is between 0.5 and 1.0. If the value is 0.5 the scores for two groups do not differ, while a score of 1.0 indicates no overlap in the distributions of the group scores (Figure 7.3). A value of 0.8 for the AUC indicates that, for 80% of the time, a random selection from the positive group will have a classifier score greater than a random selection from the negative class (Deleo, 1993). A value of 0.5 for the AUC is equivalent to selecting classes using a random event such as the result of a coin toss.

Despite its advantages, the ROC plot does not provide a rule for the classification of cases. However, there are strategies that can be used to develop decision rules from the ROC plot (Deleo, 1993; Zweig and Campbell, 1993). Finding the appropriate threshold from a ROC plot depends on having values for the relative costs of false-positive and false-negative errors. Assigning values to these costs is complex, potentially subjective and dependent upon the context within which the classification rule will be used (Section 7.8). As a guideline Zweig and Campbell (1993) suggest that if the false-positive costs (FPCs) exceed the false-negative costs (FNCs) the threshold should favour specificity, while sensitivity should be favoured if FPCs are greater than the FNCs. Combining these costs with the prevalence (p) of positive cases allows the calculation of a slope (Zweig and Campbell, 1993):

$$m = (FPC/FNC) \times ((1 - P)/P)$$

where m describes the slope of a tangent to the ROC plot if it is a smooth and parametric curve. The point at which this tangent touches the curve identifies the particular sensitivity/specificity pair that should be used to select the threshold. If the ROC plot is a stepped non-parametric curve the equivalent sensitivity/specificity pair is found by moving a line, with slope m, from the top left of the ROC plot. The sensitivity/specificity pair is located where the line and the curve first touch (Zweig and Campbell, 1993). If costs are equal FNC/FPC = 1, so m becomes the ratio of negative to positive cases with a slope of 1 for equal proportions. As the prevalence declines, m becomes increasingly steep.

7.7.3   Comparing classifiers using AUC values

ROC plots can be used to compare classifiers. If the classifiers have ROC curves, rather than single points, the area under the ROC curve (AUC) is a useful index. This is because the AUC is equal to the probability that the classifier will rank a randomly chosen positive instance higher than a randomly chosen negative instance. The AUC is also closely related to the Gini index, which is twice the area between the diagonal and the ROC curve, and the Wilcoxon test.

Because there is no reason why a ROC curve for one classifier should be consistently above or below that of another classifier over all thresholds it is possible that relative performance will change with the threshold. This is a further complication when it comes to comparing classifier performance.

It is important to remember that the classifier's performance will have been estimated using a sample of training cases. As such the AUC for one particular training set is only an estimate of the classifier's performance over all possible data. This is potentially a problem when classifiers are compared. It is not possible to compare single AUC estimates if there is no information about the expected variability over a range of different training samples. Fawcett (2003) presents details of averaging techniques that can be used to combine the results from different test sets to obtain confidence intervals for performance.

7.8   Incorporating costs

7.8.1   Costs are universal

In all binary classifiers there are two potential mistakes. If these mistakes are assumed to be equivalent the optimal rule is to assign a case to the class that has highest posterior probability, given the predictors. Typically, this will be the largest class. If the mistakes are not equivalent it is necessary to weight them (attach costs). Attaching costs to classification mistakes can be emotive, with some surprising antagonism against apparently arbitrary evaluations of relative costs. However, there are many situations in which there is an obvious inequality in relative costs. For example, in a cancer screening programme the cost of a false-negative error far exceeds that of a false-positive error. It is less clear what the relative costs should be: 1:2, 1:5, 1:10, 1:100? The only certainty is that it should not be 1:1.

In any literature review it is clear that few biological studies *explicitly* include costs in the classifier design and evaluation. However, *all* studies implicitly apply costs, even if the authors have not recognised it! This surprising statement reflects the fact that a failure to explicitly allocate costs results in the default, and least desirable, equal cost model. Unfortunately, it is impossible to provide advice on specific values for misclassification costs because these will always involve subject-specific judgements. In many respects this echoes Fisher's later view about significance levels: 'No scientific worker has a fixed level of significance from year to year, and in all circumstances, he rejects hypothesis; he rather gives his mind to each particular case in the light of his evidence and ideas' (cited in Upton, 1992, p. 397). Interestingly, Fisher originally advocated fixed significance levels unlike Pearson who advocated a significance level that provided a balance between type I and type II errors.

7.8.2   Types of cost

Turney (2000) recognised nine levels of cost in classifier design and use. The first is the most obvious category concerning the misclassification of cases. However, he breaks this down into five sub-categories: the most commonly used constant cost (a global cost for each class) model; a case-specific cost that varies between cases (for example if a class was 'extinction prone' the cost could take account of the population size for each species); a case-specific cost that depends on a value for a predictor rather than the class; a time-sensitive cost that is conditional on the time of the misclassification; and a final cost that is conditional on other errors. The other costs relate to the development of the classifier and include costs related to obtaining the data and the computational complexity. Hollmén *et al.* (2000) argue that unequal, but fixed, misclassification costs are too coarse and that costs should be calculated separately for each case.

7.8.3   Using misclassification costs

A misclassification cost is a function of the relationship between the predicted and actual class. These costs are relatively easily represented in a two-class predictor but it becomes more difficult with multi-class classifiers (see Lynn *et al.*, 1995). If costs are applied, the aim changes from one of minimising the number of errors (maximising accuracy) to one which minimises the cost of the errors. Consequently, the imposition of costs complicates how the classifier's performance should be assessed. For example, we now need to take account of the costs that could be incurred from the imposition of the trivial rule of assigning cases to the least costly class. There are different methods by which costs can be applied. Firstly, the allocation threshold can be varied (Section 7.5) so that misclassification costs are optimised. Andrews and Metton (1987) described in detail how this can be used with logistic regression. A second method uses case weights or over-sampling to make the most cost-sensitive class the majority class. In general, classifiers are more accurate with the majority class. However, the most common method, and the one that is used in most machine learning applications, is a cost matrix that weights errors prior to the calculation of model accuracy. For example, in a conservation-based model we may be able to assign weights by taking into account perceived threats to the species. However, in the absence of clear economic gains and losses, the allocation of such weights must be subjective. The cost associated with an error depends upon the relationship between the actual and allocated classes. Misclassification costs need not be reciprocal; for example classifying A as B may be more costly than classifying B as A. Lynn *et al.* (1995) used a matrix of misclassification costs to evaluate the performance of a decision-tree model for the prediction of landscape levels of potential forest vegetation. Their cost structure was based on the amount of compositional similarity between pairs of groups. It is worth noting that in the Lynn *et al.* (1995) example the classes are not discrete. This is an example of a more general, but frequently ignored, problem. It is generally assumed that classes are discrete, for example gender, and that class membership is known without error. There are many situations where this assumption is unjustified and it becomes necessary, but difficult, to incorporate this additional error into the supervised classification procedure. Obviously if classes are not defined unambiguously, it becomes more difficult to apply a classification procedure, and any measure of accuracy is likely to be compromised. This is a problem that applies equally to statistical procedures such as logistic regression (Magder and Hughes, 1997). Provost and Fawcett (1997) suggested using a ROC analysis to deal with the imprecision in class proportions and misclassification costs. Their method is similar to that suggested by Zweig and Campbell (1993) but uses a convex hull derived from two or more ROC curves, derived from classifiers that have different class or cost structures, to identify potentially optimum classifiers. Provost and Fawcett (1997) showed that the convex hull of the classifier ROC curve is the locus of optimum performance for that set of classifiers.

Remaley *et al.* (1999) described an extension to ROC plots that produces a three-dimensional, or contour, plot which combines unit cost ratios and prevalence to identify appropriate thresholds and compare classifiers. They were particularly concerned with ensuring that comparisons were made over a clinically realistic range of cost and prevalence values.

7.9   Comparing classifiers

Superficially it seems that comparing classifier performance should be simple; indeed there are many papers that compare performance within a relatively narrow biological discipline (e.g. Brosse and Lek, 2000; Dudoit *et al.*, 2002; Lee *et al.*, 2005; Manel *et al.*, 1999a,b). While these comparisons probably serve a useful purpose in the raising of awareness they sometimes oversimplify the process and generalise too much about their findings. Unfortunately it is not easy to demonstrate superiority of performance, if only because there is no single measure that should always be employed (Hand, 1997). Judging between classifiers depends on having sensible criteria and techniques for ranking their performance. Almost all classifier comparisons use overall accuracy as their metric but, as shown above, this can be unreliable. Even the more robust AUC measure can be a problem, for example when the comparison is between a stepped and a continuous ROC function.

Before beginning any comparison it is worth remembering what Wolpert and Macready (1995) said in their 'no-free-lunch' (NFL) theorem. This is a proof that there is no 'best' algorithm over all possible classification problems and they showed that, although one classifier may outperform another on problem A, it is possible that the ranking would be reversed for problem B. Indeed the NFL theorem shows that it is impossible, in the absence of prior domain knowledge, to choose between two algorithms based on their previous behaviour. The original and additional papers on this topic can be obtained from http://www.no-free-lunch.org.

Comparison of classifiers is an active area of research, and some controversy, within the machine learning community (e.g. Duin, 1996; Lim *et al.*, 2000; Mitchie *et al.*, 1994; Salzberg, 1997). The most comprehensive comparative study of a range of methods is in the book by Mitchie *et al.* (1994). This book is based on the EC (ESPRIT) project StatLog which compared and evaluated 23 classification techniques over 22 real-world data sets, including an assessment of their merits, disadvantages and application. Although it is now out of print, the authors have made it freely available in Acrobat pdf format and it is certainly worth reading if one intends to use a classifier. The main conclusion from the study was, as predicted by the NFL theorem, that there was no best classifier over the tested data sets, although the nearest-neighbour classifier and feed-forward neural networks tended to have a good performance over a range of data sets. A less intensive, but equally wide-ranging, series of comparisons was undertaken by Lim *et al.* (2000). They investigated the performance of 22 decision trees, 9 statistical and 2 neural networks over 32 data sets. They showed that there were no significant differences in accuracy across most of the algorithms and any differences were so small that they had no practical significance. Their conclusion was that the choice of classifier must be driven by factors other than accuracy. This is reasonable since the existence of the NFL theorem means that other factors, such as size of the training set, missing values and probability distributions, are likely to be more important guides to the choice of classifier algorithm. It also suggests that algorithm comparisons should be treated with caution, or at least with a recognition that the algorithm rankings are probably only applicable to the specific set of data tested.

One of the difficulties with classifier comparisons is the range of comparisons and the occasional lack of clarity in the reason for the comparison. For example, it is possible to phrase a classifier comparison within the context of different instances of one classifier, for example a logistic regression with different predictor sets or different classifiers with the same data set, or the effect of class proportions on performance, etc. The ways in which classifiers can be compared is at least partly dependent on the rationale for the comparison, while the non-independence of data sets creates statistical difficulties. In an attempt to overcome his critique of earlier comparisons Salzberg (1997) sets out a rigorous procedure that is outlined below. Salzberg's concerns arise from previous reviews of classifier comparisons. In particular he cites the extensive reviews undertaken by Prechelt (1997) and Flexer (1996) as evidence of a lack of rigour. One common problem is the lack of independence between studies that should be reflected in a correction to the value of alpha used when looking for evidence of significant differences in accuracy. He also cites the common practice of classifier 'tuning' which goes undocumented and one of his recommendations deals with the problems created by this practice. The importance of user-tuning, at least for neural networks, is also highlighted by Duin (1996). Indeed he wonders if some comparisons are more to do with the experts rather than the algorithms. Salzberg also notes that a simple comparison of overall accuracy is inadequate. Instead he suggests that the comparison should use four numbers that examine how two classifiers differ with respect to individual cases. For example, both could correctly (a) or incorrectly predict (d) the class of a case; alternatively one or other could make an incorrect prediction (b and c). The last pair of numbers can be used in a simple binomial test. Huberty (1994) describes how a test must compare if $(a + b)/(a + b + c + d)$ is significantly different from $(a + c)/(a + b + c + d)$. Huberty (1994) suggests using McNemar's test to calculate $(b - c)^2/(b + c)$, which has an approximate chi-squared value with one degree of freedom when $b + c$ is 'large'. Multiple comparisons can be carried out using Cochran's Q test. Huberty (1994) has additional details.

Salzberg's suggested approach begins with the choice of a test data set. Ideally, this should be capable of illustrating the new classifier's strengths, for example the ability to handle a large number of predictors. This should then be split into k segments (normally $k = 10$). Each segment is withheld, in turn, while the remaining data are split into a tuning and training segment. The tuning segment is used to set the classifier's parameters (e.g. size of the hidden layer in a neural network) while the training segment is used to derive the classifier (e.g. setting the weights in a neural network). The trained network is then tested on the withheld kth segment. This is repeated for each withheld segment and the classifier's mean accuracy and variance is derived from the k accuracy measures. Classifiers can also be compared using the binomial test or McNemar's test of agreement.

Duin (1996) also makes an important point about the role of a designer that needs to be considered when comparing classifiers. Some require extensive tuning by an expert, a feature that can be seen as both an advantage and a disadvantage. Other classifiers require very little tuning and are essentially automatic. Again this can be viewed as an advantage or disadvantage. He suggests that it is difficult to compare these two groups in an objective way.

7.10   Recommended reading

It should now be obvious that measuring accuracy, and comparing classifiers, is not as simple as we might hope. Fortunately there are some good resources that provide general or subject-specific advice on appropriate methods. Undoubtedly the ROC plot is identified by most as the 'best' method, although it is also important to recognise the role that bias and variance play in assessing the quality of an accuracy estimate. Fawcett's (2002) review of ROC plots is one of the best, and most accessible, accounts of the theory and practice of using the method to assess accuracy. In addition, Swets *et al.* (2000) wrote a popular review of decision making that emphasised the value of ROC plots. Hand's (1997) book is a well-written and authoritative account that links the design of classifiers to their assessment. Altman and Royston's (2000) thoughtful review of model validation, in a clinical context, raises some important issues that will benefit the wider biological community. Finally, Baldi *et al.* (2000) and Fielding and Bell (1997) wrote review articles that discuss approaches to accuracy assessment in protein secondary structure prediction and ecological presence/absence modelling. Fielding (1999b, 2002) also extended his ideas with respect to ecological models.

Appendix A

PCA data set 1

A.1 Outline

This is an artificial data set that was created with a known correlation structure. There are 5 variables and 30 cases. The variables fall into two related (correlated groups), hence the effective dimensions of these data are 30 by 2.

A.2 The data

A.2.1 Descriptive statistics and relationships between variables

There are two obvious points to draw from these simple summary statistics. Firstly, V2 has a much larger mean than any of the other variables. Secondly, although V4 has a relatively large mean, its standard deviation is small, since most of the other variables have standard deviations that are about 50% of the mean.

There are two major groups of correlated predictors in Figure A.1 and Table A.3. The first three variables, V1–V3, are quite highly inter-correlated, particularly V2 and V3. V4 and V5 are also correlated. The only other significant relationship is the weak, negative correlation between V1 and V5.

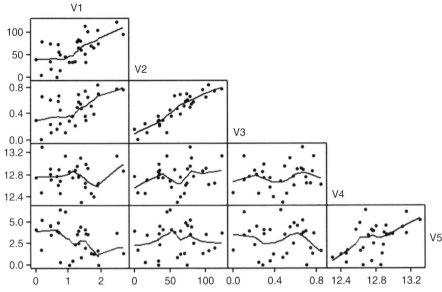

Figure A.1 Scatter plot matrix, with loess smoother lines, of the five variables V1–V5.

Table A.1. *The individual values*

V1	V2	V3	V4	V5
1.53	114.01	0.75	12.65	1.96
0.18	79.53	0.67	13.30	5.28
1.90	105.63	0.85	12.62	1.71
0.91	45.62	0.11	13.14	6.24
1.27	79.48	0.50	12.95	3.61
1.52	52.08	0.36	12.57	4.10
1.32	83.87	0.58	12.77	2.53
1.04	33.94	0.29	12.85	0.04
0.70	72.94	0.59	12.61	4.94
1.54	34.22	0.30	12.99	3.66
0.75	50.39	0.46	12.68	6.45
1.22	35.04	0.21	12.88	2.42
1.31	65.25	0.70	12.76	3.98
0.64	0.00	0.16	12.77	3.96
0.00	39.65	0.30	12.75	4.12
1.93	74.27	0.71	12.65	0.00
2.70	96.93	0.77	12.87	1.32
1.78	65.29	0.39	12.40	1.25
1.71	70.57	0.52	12.46	1.36

Table A.1. (cont.)

V1	V2	V3	V4	V5
0.44	75.09	0.62	12.91	4.63
2.49	124.00	0.78	13.14	3.71
1.61	101.89	0.66	12.92	3.57
0.75	15.26	0.25	12.46	0.31
0.17	5.05	0.00	12.47	1.74
1.13	33.39	0.36	12.75	0.46
1.38	81.35	0.55	13.10	4.49
0.44	34.97	0.23	12.80	4.52
0.47	17.89	0.11	12.71	3.53
1.40	60.57	0.48	12.30	0.92
0.71	56.68	0.68	12.89	3.79

Table A.2. *Descriptive statistics for the five variables V1–V5*

Variable	Range	Minimum	Maximum	Mean	Standard deviation
V1	2.70	0.00	2.70	1.166	0.660
V2	124.00	0.00	124.00	60.160	31.758
V3	0.85	0.00	0.85	0.464	0.232
V4	1.00	12.30	13.30	12.771	0.235
V5	6.45	0.00	6.45	3.020	1.806

Table A.3. *Correlation coefficients between the five variables V1–V5. Figures below the correlation coefficients are two-tailed p values. For example, the correlation between V2 and V3 is 0.895 with a p value of 0.000 and the correlation between V1 and V4 is −0.030 with a p value of 0.877*

	V1	V2	V3	V4
V2	0.631			
	0.000			
V3	0.555	0.895		
	0.001	0.000		
V4	−0.030	0.244	0.163	
	0.877	0.193	0.390	
V5	−0.399	0.032	−0.045	0.533
	0.029	0.867	0.812	0.002

Appendix B

Stickleback behaviour

B.1   Outline

The source of these data is unknown. I would be very happy to acknowledge the source once it is known. There are 7 variables and 54 cases. These data (Tables B.1 and B.2) relate to an experiment investigating the behaviour of male stickleback. The responses of male fish during an observation period were recorded, these included the response to a 'model' male fish.

B.2   The data

B.2.1   *Descriptive statistics and relationships between variables*

The large standard deviations, relative to the means (Table B.3), suggest that some of these variables do not have symmetrical frequency distributions. Apart from bites and lunges few of the variables have large correlations (Table B.4) and some of the relationships (Figure B.1) do not look monotonic. It is possible that some of the significant correlations are artefacts or possibly spurious.

Table B.1. *Variable descriptions*

Variable	Notes
LUNGES	The number of lunges towards the model male.
BITES	The number of times that the male model was bitten.
ZIGZAGS	The 'zig-zag' display is part of display behaviour, designed to attract females.
NEST	The number of nest building behaviours.
SPINES	The number of times the fish raised the 'spines' on its back.
DNEST	The duration of nest building activities.
BOUT	The number of 'bout-facing' behaviours (male–male interaction).

Table B.2. *Individual values for the seven variables*

LUNGES	BITES	ZIGZAGS	NEST	SPINES	DNEST	BOUT
79	25	0	0	15	0	45
136	58	6	0	15	0	148
115	30	2	1	9	5	29
129	139	16	0	22	0	69
120	58	15	15	14	82	9
217	78	13	1	28	3	57
173	175	3	0	46	0	73
119	65	25	1	5	3	10
174	115	4	0	14	0	304
67	34	8	2	14	117	23
87	50	6	1	28	8	21
121	67	26	1	5	0	23
177	115	4	0	14	0	305
147	25	5	0	14	0	16
67	35	21	5	24	108	9
85	35	4	0	16	0	30
81	17	0	0	16	0	43
118	30	2	1	11	1	28
277	157	2	1	12	23	47
140	134	0	0	17	0	147
71	31	9	2	14	114	25
143	54	1	0	6	0	7
143	139	16	0	22	0	72
169	169	3	0	46	0	73
143	133	0	1	16	64	133
60	5	10	0	19	0	306
157	74	5	0	18	0	302
121	76	17	0	25	0	101

Table B.2. (cont.)

LUNGES	BITES	ZIGZAGS	NEST	SPINES	DNEST	BOUT
116	61	2	0	26	0	45
159	82	4	0	17	0	298
120	85	7	3	31	122	23
67	34	21	5	25	102	28
208	59	4	1	18	133	297
156	25	4	1	13	76	6
165	102	3	0	16	0	77
137	55	2	3	7	199	8
277	152	3	1	11	19	49
147	70	7	0	11	0	153
130	69	11	0	27	0	31
142	73	7	0	12	0	158
211	80	14	1	28	2	42
132	55	6	0	14	0	152
42	4	1	2	10	136	33
108	59	1	0	28	0	41
83	30	3	4	15	177	49
125	67	11	0	23	0	36
64	11	10	0	20	0	306
117	94	7	3	31	125	20
117	54	15	15	14	85	12
124	72	17	4	25	146	78
160	108	1	0	15	0	87
204	57	4	0	17	0	303
41	3	0	0	9	0	30
96	45	5	2	27	0	6

Table B.3. *Descriptive statistics for the seven variables*

Variable	Minimum	Maximum	Mean	Standard deviation
LUNGES	41	277	131.19	50.77
BITES	3	175	69.06	43.43
ZIGZAGS	0	26	7.28	6.69
NEST	0	15	1.43	3.00
SPINES	5	46	18.43	8.71
DNEST	0	199	34.26	56.49
BOUT	6	306	89.31	98.68

Table B.4. *Correlation coefficients between the seven variables. Figures below the correlation coefficients are two-tailed* p *values. For example, the correlation between LUNGES and ZIGZAGS is* −0.139 *with a* p *value of 0.315*

	LUNGES	BITES	ZIGZAGS	NEST	SPINES	DNEST
BITES	0.688					
	0.000					
ZIGZAGS	−0.139	−0.043				
	0.315	0.759				
NEST	−0.164	−0.149	0.352			
	0.236	0.283	0.009			
SPINES	0.056	0.373	0.068	−0.053		
	0.690	0.005	0.626	0.706		
DNEST	−0.229	−0.218	0.091	0.514	−0.051	
	0.096	0.114	0.511	0.000	0.714	
BOUT	0.233	0.117	−0.161	−0.306	−0.041	−0.242
	0.090	0.398	0.246	0.024	0.766	0.078

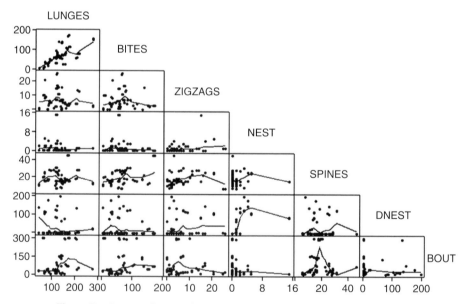

Figure B.1 Scatter plot matrix, with loess smoother lines, of the seven variables.

Appendix C

Bacterial data

C.1 Outline

The data (Table C.1) are part of a data set described by Rataj and Schindler (1991). Data are presented for 6 species, most having data for more than 1 strain and 16 phenotypic characters (0 = absent, 1 = present). The species are: *Escherichia coli* (ecoli), *Salmonella typhi* (styphi), *Klebsiella pneumoniae* (kpneu), *Proteus vulgaris* (pvul), *P. morganii* (pmor) and *Serratia marcescens* (smar).

Table C.1. *Presence (1) or absence (0) of 16 phenotypic traits in samples of bacteria*

Taxon	H2S	MAN	LYS	IND	ORN	CIT	URE	ONP	VPT	INO	LIP	PHE	MAL	ADO	ARA	RHA
ecoli1	0	1	1	1	0	0	0	1	0	0	0	0	0	0	1	1
ecoli2	0	1	0	1	1	0	0	1	0	0	0	0	0	0	1	0
ecoli3	1	1	0	1	1	0	0	1	0	0	0	0	0	0	1	1
styphi1	0	1	1	0	0	0	0	0	0	0	0	0	0	0	1	0
styphi2	0	1	1	0	0	0	0	0	0	0	0	0	0	0	0	0
styphi3	1	1	1	0	0	0	0	0	0	0	0	0	0	0	1	0
kpneu1	0	1	1	1	0	1	1	1	1	1	0	0	0	1	1	1
kpneu2	0	1	1	1	0	1	1	1	1	1	0	0	1	0	1	1
kpneu3	0	1	1	1	0	1	1	1	1	1	0	0	1	1	1	1
kpneu4	0	1	1	1	0	1	1	1	0	1	0	0	1	1	1	1
kpncu5	0	1	1	1	0	1	0	1	1	1	0	0	1	1	1	1
pvul1	1	0	0	1	0	1	1	0	0	0	0	1	0	0	0	0
pvul2	1	0	0	1	0	0	0	0	0	0	0	1	0	0	0	0
pvul3	1	0	0	1	0	0	1	0	0	0	0	1	0	0	0	0
pmor1	0	0	1	1	1	0	1	0	0	0	0	1	0	0	0	0
pmor2	0	0	0	1	1	0	0	0	0	0	0	1	0	0	0	0
smar	0	1	1	0	1	1	0	1	1	0	1	0	0	0	0	0

Appendix D

The human genus

D.1   Outline

This analysis uses data (Table D.1) extracted from Table 5 in Wood and Collard (1999). There are 12 gnathic variables from 8 taxa related to the present day *Homo sapiens*. Wood and Collard conclude that *H. habilis* and *H. rudolfensis* do not belong in the genus and that the earliest taxa to satisfy the criteria are *H. ergaster* or early African *H. erectus*. The other genera are *Paranthropus* and *Australopithecus*.

D.2   The data

D.2.1   Descriptive statistics and relationships between variables

It is very clear from Figure D.1 that most of the variables are highly correlated and contribute little independent information. If the data are subjected to a principal components analysis 89% of the variance is retained in the first component, whose eigen value is 9.76. The second component, with an eigen value of 0.87, retains a further 7.9% of the variance giving a total of 96.6% for the first two components.

Table D.1. *Hominin species means for 11 gnathic variables. The variables are (1) symphyseal height, (2) symphyseal breadth, (3) corpus height at M1, (4) corpus width at M1, (5) P4 mesiodistal diameter, (6) P4 buccolingual diameter, (7) M1 mesiodistal diameter, (8) M1 buccolingual diameter, (9) M2 mesiodistal diameter, (10) M2 buccolingual diameter, and (11) M3 area. Data from Table 5 in Wood and Collard (1999)*

Taxon	1	2	3	4	5	6	7	8	9	10	11
A. africanus	41	20	33	23	9.3	11.0	13.2	12.9	14.9	14.1	218
P. boisei	51	29	42	29	14.2	15.5	16.7	15.7	20.4	18.5	327
P. robustus	50	28	39	27	11.7	14.0	15.1	14.1	16.6	15.7	254
H. erectus	37	19	36	22	8.9	11.3	12.4	12.0	13.3	12.7	145
H. ergaster	33	20	31	19	8.7	11.0	13.1	11.6	13.8	12.3	170
H. habilis	27	19	29	21	9.8	10.5	13.9	12.3	14.9	12.6	201
H. neanderthalensis	42	15	34	18	7.1	8.7	10.6	10.7	11.1	10.7	131
H. rudolfensis	36	23	36	23	10.5	12.0	14.0	13.2	16.4	13.7	250
H. sapiens	34	14	29	13	7.1	8.4	11.2	10.5	10.8	10.5	113

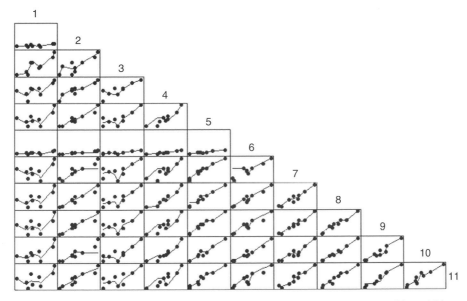

Figure D.1 Scatter plot matrix, with loess smoother lines, of the 11 gnathic variables. Axis values are not shown.

Appendix E

Artificial data set with two correlation patterns

E.1   Outline

There are two data sets (Table E.1) that differ in the amount of correlation. Each data set has four predictors, a1–a4 and b1–b4, and there is a class variable that is common to both. The predictors a1–a4 are uncorrelated with each other while there are some correlations within data set B.

E.2   The data

E.2.1   Descriptive statistics and relationships between variables

Both data sets show a trend of increasing means across both classes that is matched by a similar increase in the standard errors (Table E.2). Table E.3 and Figure E.1 clearly show the different correlation structures within the two data sets. There are no significant between-predictor correlations in data set A. However, in data set B b3 and b4 are highly correlated, although all other between-predictor correlations are insignificant.

Table E.1. *Two groups of potential predictors (a1–a4 and b1–b4) plus a shared class variable*

Class	a1	a2	a3	a4	b1	b2	b3	b4
0	8.20	20.10	18.06	15.46	10.65	16.92	19.79	20.63
0	10.80	14.10	22.78	30.58	6.07	11.00	15.31	12.46
0	10.96	18.30	20.80	23.91	11.05	8.11	22.63	28.73
0	11.62	14.82	22.69	26.90	9.60	20.60	23.42	24.16
0	10.00	15.05	24.80	29.90	10.23	15.77	15.70	27.72
0	10.55	20.06	21.63	30.13	14.40	13.98	19.74	19.80
0	9.69	14.96	21.49	26.35	8.70	14.76	25.74	32.14
0	11.62	13.99	21.02	30.00	10.14	14.91	18.58	20.34
0	8.48	13.89	25.40	25.26	6.90	16.27	22.88	19.60
0	9.35	13.32	24.20	22.58	10.57	16.05	16.77	23.60
0	11.33	15.50	19.19	31.06	10.57	20.70	17.83	23.75
0	14.06	11.40	17.92	5.90	8.80	24.10	19.51	17.89
0	11.42	16.36	18.33	19.31	11.90	17.81	17.50	30.76
0	12.12	16.92	19.21	29.27	15.70	13.33	19.24	22.01
0	10.80	8.08	20.96	26.64	9.84	14.25	20.50	19.09
0	8.57	16.64	23.62	26.72	8.20	18.66	18.70	26.03
0	11.81	16.30	17.67	27.52	9.28	15.69	22.93	19.59
0	9.73	16.51	17.22	29.55	10.50	17.11	21.98	21.31
0	6.19	17.20	15.60	29.80	6.54	13.14	22.29	25.18
0	11.64	13.69	25.15	8.70	9.49	11.18	18.84	23.58
0	11.55	9.21	17.77	29.92	9.09	25.80	23.32	30.87
0	10.19	16.35	18.76	33.66	9.30	16.95	21.82	27.21
0	7.48	12.51	21.51	32.70	9.88	14.47	20.88	30.06
0	10.86	9.50	23.84	19.68	7.90	11.55	24.22	25.22
0	10.31	15.60	22.24	23.96	8.80	13.86	24.49	30.45
0	11.00	15.73	17.45	19.80	6.31	17.87	15.36	23.02
0	13.01	17.02	22.14	23.25	11.95	12.16	18.66	24.97
0	8.67	12.67	21.60	26.66	5.88	18.36	21.38	30.34
0	8.43	13.67	17.44	31.70	11.40	7.33	22.04	29.74
0	9.35	14.27	16.90	25.90	11.58	16.69	15.92	22.09
0	10.77	14.92	16.30	22.15	8.48	13.56	15.90	27.50
0	11.35	14.03	19.99	27.00	10.35	16.62	14.86	10.07
0	11.64	17.85	22.86	23.90	8.72	18.89	22.10	30.25
0	11.67	17.43	26.01	22.55	9.49	19.18	24.73	31.22
0	11.20	21.95	25.02	25.80	9.50	10.81	22.18	39.26
0	12.29	16.91	19.98	25.90	11.24	15.06	21.00	23.95
0	8.80	16.40	19.46	22.00	9.50	8.98	22.29	21.49
0	12.09	15.59	17.20	28.50	9.50	17.44	18.50	25.16
0	8.12	16.42	30.05	24.01	10.89	16.41	19.49	29.07
0	10.53	12.50	22.56	21.75	15.70	8.50	20.03	24.14

Table E.1. (cont.)

Class	a1	a2	a3	a4	b1	b2	b3	b4
0	10.04	18.16	18.29	24.33	10.32	16.25	11.98	15.32
0	9.63	13.06	23.67	19.40	8.67	16.57	18.54	27.33
0	10.84	14.49	23.01	23.51	10.05	18.01	20.58	29.28
0	9.21	11.65	27.61	28.42	11.93	17.43	23.26	24.51
0	12.68	11.20	16.86	21.78	11.05	14.20	18.22	12.82
0	11.02	14.07	18.10	28.92	9.81	17.48	24.27	36.78
0	6.55	14.69	13.79	37.70	8.30	14.61	15.52	22.67
0	7.78	12.36	22.06	25.64	11.10	16.07	19.00	21.94
0	8.56	17.10	22.52	21.99	9.57	13.77	24.20	30.60
0	9.92	16.31	24.48	24.67	13.70	12.90	24.20	35.19
0	11.21	14.30	20.30	30.29	9.82	14.31	18.38	29.62
0	10.43	14.20	16.60	27.95	9.93	18.40	20.57	26.98
0	9.48	12.93	20.40	24.03	9.65	12.62	17.49	29.94
0	12.40	15.61	21.40	27.49	7.50	14.40	16.37	12.70
0	12.28	16.60	22.31	34.60	10.27	17.53	16.68	22.66
0	9.99	13.55	16.49	20.73	10.44	11.73	25.21	38.86
0	10.50	15.80	18.36	19.39	10.20	12.05	16.75	27.34
0	9.67	13.31	21.20	21.49	10.40	11.00	26.44	26.55
0	4.87	15.15	21.80	26.82	6.74	14.21	14.51	8.47
0	4.58	12.16	15.50	27.70	13.60	16.70	24.50	39.11
0	6.41	20.56	16.12	24.70	9.04	15.59	27.39	29.34
0	5.71	14.69	24.89	21.55	9.76	10.67	21.66	36.74
0	9.60	10.97	22.10	25.64	7.80	19.47	20.42	17.29
0	9.79	16.36	23.66	26.50	7.83	15.01	25.44	25.56
0	9.36	18.70	18.52	17.17	10.11	16.11	20.97	23.87
0	10.16	18.31	16.60	30.05	11.20	16.55	20.25	23.05
0	9.04	21.54	20.46	29.75	10.15	15.20	26.96	36.91
0	10.65	14.84	21.01	18.47	11.46	11.83	27.44	27.96
0	9.37	15.12	25.10	27.44	8.83	10.58	19.79	26.45
0	3.48	15.27	17.99	26.40	9.09	15.40	19.47	22.32
0	7.72	14.98	16.49	24.24	10.22	13.36	20.38	29.13
0	9.02	10.97	20.48	17.59	6.74	13.30	20.30	28.68
0	9.93	14.77	27.36	22.84	8.67	15.22	14.61	14.74
0	6.80	18.58	17.97	19.90	9.06	14.45	20.90	23.63
0	9.39	20.51	21.30	23.73	9.05	9.80	22.03	27.10
1	14.62	22.40	28.81	32.91	9.85	15.10	29.57	44.62
1	7.85	20.61	25.40	29.48	14.02	14.63	30.00	32.66
1	13.57	18.65	23.71	32.48	15.23	19.06	20.03	35.93
1	8.41	12.06	27.10	28.93	12.19	12.37	32.06	37.21
1	10.60	15.75	25.51	24.56	13.09	23.57	31.36	35.74
1	12.58	19.95	16.84	33.79	9.90	13.74	26.34	28.96

Table E.1. (cont.)

Class	a1	a2	a3	a4	b1	b2	b3	b4
1	11.66	16.78	28.50	25.90	10.37	16.65	26.25	31.21
1	11.86	17.07	19.75	20.57	9.27	19.47	19.92	26.46
1	12.55	19.22	27.75	37.00	8.90	19.00	24.73	29.82
1	9.71	20.70	20.33	21.91	11.60	23.39	22.54	19.74
1	8.59	23.92	23.10	25.21	10.51	8.58	25.63	22.71
1	10.80	16.54	27.14	24.07	14.20	19.26	16.20	19.94
1	7.61	18.86	23.03	30.17	9.80	24.87	17.04	21.08
1	12.40	17.40	27.90	39.57	15.30	19.19	29.55	52.70
1	12.52	14.56	23.76	28.59	12.68	11.90	20.90	21.42
1	8.55	14.09	24.66	22.88	9.80	15.40	24.00	18.30
1	8.27	18.34	20.73	26.67	10.10	17.01	21.24	18.73
1	11.50	15.89	25.86	27.63	12.48	26.92	26.00	33.49
1	11.31	19.85	26.44	34.74	15.14	15.72	16.16	10.37
1	11.47	18.15	29.29	33.63	17.92	20.45	16.04	23.98
1	14.50	14.05	22.98	26.01	9.57	20.52	23.76	22.05
1	14.50	18.06	22.60	27.10	8.68	19.42	25.21	31.51
1	14.08	21.02	26.67	40.70	14.85	20.87	22.84	28.80
1	14.74	26.55	23.10	30.42	13.33	19.34	32.53	34.37
1	13.74	17.76	26.90	34.51	14.34	20.97	26.41	36.11
1	7.00	18.61	26.20	30.60	13.71	20.09	26.38	34.40
1	11.86	15.32	21.97	26.43	12.70	17.62	26.66	18.86
1	11.52	12.92	27.51	20.36	9.58	21.05	27.68	24.50
1	9.70	21.73	22.60	33.57	14.70	17.50	24.48	28.76
1	13.84	21.85	30.00	22.71	7.84	18.29	27.86	36.89
1	10.10	15.77	22.77	22.82	12.26	25.76	27.98	38.45
1	7.87	20.08	25.61	22.69	12.38	19.47	22.94	24.22
1	11.10	17.57	25.85	37.40	10.14	18.51	17.10	22.23
1	12.45	17.74	19.26	30.89	13.42	13.96	20.48	16.90
1	9.79	20.79	25.88	23.90	9.09	14.56	19.09	20.54
1	8.74	15.51	25.51	38.90	12.31	17.25	27.92	43.46
1	11.55	12.84	26.35	28.11	8.90	16.96	24.23	33.59
1	7.91	16.60	32.49	31.37	12.60	12.46	30.94	33.53
1	10.46	26.14	19.97	27.12	13.20	16.19	23.61	24.99
1	12.42	17.54	26.00	35.57	7.71	20.97	21.91	20.77
1	12.81	9.57	20.21	36.26	8.81	17.63	13.35	10.90
1	9.67	17.99	26.00	23.02	14.30	15.83	30.66	34.90
1	13.28	22.66	23.10	6.60	11.31	19.33	24.69	44.91
1	14.15	11.43	23.50	20.70	9.23	15.73	27.63	27.52
1	6.41	18.11	25.03	22.76	12.31	20.78	29.10	38.20
1	12.97	15.59	18.62	28.39	13.39	23.62	28.50	37.50
1	9.80	19.05	24.15	28.34	12.22	17.31	14.47	27.31

Table E.1. (cont.)

Class	a1	a2	a3	a4	b1	b2	b3	b4
1	9.86	21.68	16.80	31.70	14.16	18.37	20.20	24.42
1	15.12	16.99	8.20	29.47	11.99	24.56	17.91	21.29
1	16.49	20.20	24.23	33.31	12.35	17.22	23.71	31.98
1	12.33	21.19	32.21	26.50	12.43	20.97	15.62	11.83
1	7.58	26.30	32.66	23.61	10.32	17.42	21.89	28.98
1	15.17	16.40	9.20	31.61	16.15	15.22	22.66	30.46
1	14.39	21.85	26.51	6.80	9.66	15.61	25.17	35.10
1	11.43	13.02	27.32	26.77	12.94	16.57	25.15	35.94
1	12.03	26.55	18.44	42.97	13.50	19.09	21.86	24.30
1	14.82	16.80	27.08	23.10	13.70	19.91	24.21	28.40
1	12.63	17.54	23.69	30.30	12.46	14.44	27.40	27.82
1	16.26	11.70	26.80	31.27	13.65	16.70	31.62	42.53
1	6.96	15.68	24.39	27.55	12.40	16.87	14.54	22.72
1	13.65	21.78	17.52	26.64	11.56	19.93	27.21	35.20
1	12.99	15.32	29.73	31.34	6.63	21.68	28.73	31.91
1	15.14	10.80	27.40	37.64	14.02	15.70	24.84	24.02
1	14.73	22.50	23.37	38.24	9.90	18.04	23.53	32.06
1	9.85	19.19	27.53	35.65	7.00	16.59	25.09	32.56
1	15.88	13.40	31.15	33.34	13.29	14.67	20.24	24.11
1	10.49	18.30	16.20	39.45	15.18	18.99	27.85	22.74
1	13.16	14.66	24.29	21.10	9.38	14.90	29.91	43.07
1	12.23	18.28	26.17	30.95	12.78	19.60	18.90	21.98
1	8.89	18.58	27.52	37.20	7.64	18.53	27.17	31.94
1	12.17	20.90	22.02	28.73	10.51	16.37	31.32	38.63
1	11.88	19.53	22.89	28.25	9.00	19.57	31.78	37.16
1	16.20	7.90	26.89	24.92	13.84	18.64	18.41	10.24
1	14.21	16.25	8.80	38.61	12.59	14.90	30.72	32.93
1	15.65	17.12	30.55	25.32	11.61	16.87	31.56	38.41

Table E.2. *Means (first two rows) and standard errors (lower two rows) for eight predictors and two classes.* n = *75 for both classes*

Class	a1	a2	a3	a4	b1	b2	b3	b4
0	9.82	15.21	20.69	25.06	9.82	15.03	20.45	25.41
1	11.81	17.92	24.21	29.07	11.81	18.08	24.44	29.12
0	0.23	0.32	0.38	0.60	0.22	0.39	0.39	0.75
1	0.30	0.44	0.56	0.77	0.27	0.38	0.57	1.00

Table E.3. *Correlation matrices for data sets A and B. The upper figure for each combination is the correlation coefficient, the lower figure is the two-tailed* p *value*

	a1	a2	a3		b1	b2	b3
a2	0.034			b2	0.127		
p	0.676			*p*	0.122		
a3	0.116	0.093		b3	0.156	0.099	
p	0.157	0.260		*p*	0.056	0.227	
a4	0.119	0.147	0.026	b4	0.145	0.074	0.700
p	0.146	0.073	0.756	*p*	0.076	0.366	0.000

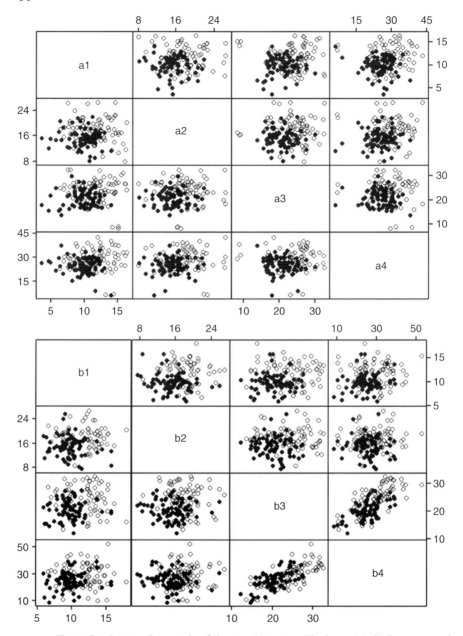

Figure E.1 Scatter plot matrix of the two data sets with classes labelled as open and filled points.

Appendix F

Regional characteristics of golden eagle ranges

F.1   Outline

These data (Table F.1) are part of a larger data set used by Fielding and Haworth (1995) to investigate the performance of bird-habitat models. They relate to the core area, the region close to the nest, of golden eagle *Aquila chrysaetos*, in three regions of western Scotland. Eight habitat variables were measured for each range. The values are the numbers of four-hectare grid cells covered by the habitat.

F.2   The data

F.2.1   *Descriptive statistics*

The box plots in Figure F.1 indicate that most of the variables, within the regions, have reasonably symmetric frequency distributions, although region two in particular has a number of unusual values (outliers). There are obvious differences between the regions for all eight variables.

Table F.1. *Habitat means for eight habitat variables. The variables are POST (mature planted conifer forest in which the tree canopy has closed); PRE (pre-canopy closure planted conifer forest); BOG (flat waterlogged land); CALL (*Calluna *(heather) heathland); WET (wet heath, mainly purple moor grass); STEEP (steeply sloping land); LT200 (land below 200 m); and L4_600 (land between 200 and 400 m)*

Region	POST	PRE	BOG	CALL	WET	STEEP	LT200	L4_600
1	0.3	2.7	18.0	2.0	0.0	3.2	0.0	4.2
1	0.8	2.2	11.1	1.3	0.0	6.3	8.3	0.3
1	3.3	4.1	14.1	0.2	0.0	4.7	1.3	4.0
1	2.7	5.6	10.6	1.3	0.0	6.1	6.6	0.3
1	0.3	1.3	14.2	0.0	0.0	3.6	4.7	14.5
1	0.8	4.0	11.0	0.4	0.0	3.8	10.1	1.5
1	3.9	6.1	13.1	0.2	0.0	2.8	0.2	8.0
2	0.0	0.0	8.4	1.9	9.9	9.1	9.1	2.0
2	0.0	7.5	5.5	0.0	9.7	8.4	16.7	0.8
2	0.0	0.0	8.8	2.7	3.8	7.8	14.0	0.9
2	8.9	0.0	8.4	2.3	5.9	7.7	9.6	3.5
2	0.0	0.0	3.7	1.0	9.2	4.7	14.2	0.6
2	0.0	0.0	1.1	0.0	11.6	20.0	1.6	10.0
2	0.3	0.0	1.0	3.0	6.6	9.9	15.8	3.4
2	0.1	1.1	6.9	0.7	6.3	5.5	16.1	0.3
2	0.0	0.0	2.3	0.6	8.3	17.4	6.4	8.3
2	0.3	4.5	0.3	0.1	3.1	15.9	7.8	7.9
2	4.9	0.3	3.4	0.5	9.4	7.1	10.5	4.8
2	0.3	0.0	3.4	0.5	4.7	0.6	23.4	0.0
2	0.0	0.0	5.5	7.1	4.7	6.0	15.3	0.0
2	0.0	0.0	6.2	8.0	1.6	5.9	15.0	0.0
2	0.0	0.0	2.1	1.5	10.3	10.8	15.9	2.5
2	0.1	0.1	5.3	2.2	12.9	12.1	6.7	5.8
3	0.0	0.0	7.9	4.6	0.0	1.2	25.0	0.0
3	0.1	0.0	8.4	7.7	0.0	2.2	25.0	0.0
3	2.9	3.3	4.8	3.4	0.0	1.4	22.9	0.0
3	0.0	10.7	7.9	1.0	0.2	1.9	22.1	0.0
3	1.1	1.8	9.6	3.0	1.4	3.2	18.1	0.0
3	1.2	1.8	15.6	1.1	1.9	2.9	12.7	0.0
3	0.0	0.0	3.7	6.8	1.6	1.8	23.0	0.0
3	0.4	0.1	13.5	3.5	2.0	2.6	11.9	0.1
3	4.9	8.1	4.0	0.2	1.0	0.9	21.6	0.0
3	0.0	0.0	12.9	3.2	1.7	1.7	21.7	0.0
3	1.4	0.0	9.8	3.8	1.1	1.9	19.2	0.0
3	0.7	0.0	13.4	3.5	3.3	2.5	11.9	0.0
3	5.6	0.8	10.3	1.3	3.0	3.0	18.9	0.0

Table F.1. (cont.)

Region	POST	PRE	BOG	CALL	WET	STEEP	LT200	L4_600
3	7.5	1.6	8.1	0.4	2.6	1.7	17.8	0.1
3	6.6	2.3	9.5	2.8	1.6	1.4	18.6	0.0
3	6.7	0.4	1.8	0.8	1.0	0.3	24.0	0.0
3	7.2	2.8	6.3	3.0	3.2	1.4	23.5	0.0

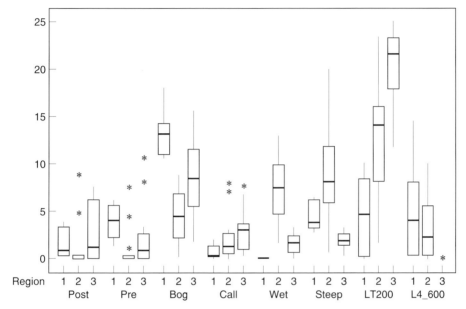

Figure F.1 Box and whisker plot of the eight habitat variables broken down by region. Outliers are mark by asterisks.

Appendix G

Characteristics of a sample of smokers and non-smokers

G.1 Outline

These data (Table G.1) are part of a data set collected by Jenkins (1991). They are simple measures and attributes recorded from a sample of 87 adults. They are used in this book to discover if a person's smoking habits can be predicted from three continuous, and two categorical, predictors. The continuous predictors are white blood cell count (wbc; $\times 10^9$ l^{-1}), body mass index (bmi; kg m^{-2}) and age (years). The two categorical predictors are gender and ABO blood type. The class variable is a binary indicator of a person's smoking habits (Y or N). The quantity of tobacco products used by each person was not recorded.

G.2 The data

G.2.1 Descriptive statistics and relationships between variables

None of the continuous predictors are correlated with each other, either overall or within the smoking groups. Neither of the categorical predictors is significantly associated with a person's smoking habits (chi-square analysis). In addition, there is no significant association between gender and blood group. White blood cell count and body mass index both differ significantly between the two smoking classes. The white blood cell count is higher in the non-smokers but the body mass index is lower. However, if a correction is applied to the p value for multiple testing the difference in body mass indices becomes insignificant. The mean ages are very similar in the two groups.

Table G.1. *Individual values for three continuous and two categorical variables for the prediction of smoking habits*

Smoke	wbc	bmi	Age	Sex	Blood group
N	5.6	28.6	43	F	AB
N	8.1	27.5	42	F	A
N	6.8	27.2	25	M	AB
N	7.3	26.6	48	F	A
N	9.0	27.2	33	F	A
N	6.4	26.4	37	F	A
Y	5.6	23.8	43	F	A
N	6.2	33.2	40	F	A
N	7.3	24.9	21	F	A
N	4.1	25.7	51	F	B
N	5.6	31.9	29	F	B
N	8.4	33.8	37	F	B
Y	5.2	26.4	44	F	B
Y	7.1	22.3	30	F	B
N	5.4	38.9	36	F	B
N	4.5	28.0	19	F	B
N	6.9	21.9	24	F	O
N	9.0	25.5	27	F	O
N	4.0	25.7	35	F	O
N	5.5	36.3	30	F	O
N	6.3	20.0	31	F	O
N	5.1	21.9	26	F	O
N	5.1	21.6	30	F	O
Y	8.4	29.0	30	F	O
N	6.0	23.1	41	F	O
N	5.6	31.4	41	F	AB
N	8.4	26.4	35	F	AB
N	5.5	24.3	20	F	AB
N	9.1	24.8	33	F	AB
N	7.1	23.2	28	F	AB
Y	8.8	28.6	33	F	AB
N	7.0	26.8	22	F	AB
Y	9.9	31.6	28	F	AB
N	7.8	25.8	37	F	AB
N	6.3	27.4	35	M	A
N	4.8	33.2	25	M	A
N	6.5	27.1	36	M	A
Y	7.4	25.6	43	M	A
N	4.6	25.9	38	M	A
N	4.7	27.7	40	M	A

Table G.1. (cont.)

Smoke	wbc	bmi	Age	Sex	Blood group
N	4.1	26.4	43	M	A
Y	4.9	29.5	34	M	A
N	2.2	26.4	21	M	A
N	5.9	32.1	34	M	A
N	5.8	28.7	28	M	A
N	6.9	27.0	33	M	A
N	4.9	25.4	33	M	A
Y	4.7	24.6	32	M	A
N	6.0	28.7	38	M	B
Y	7.4	21.9	22	M	B
N	5.4	18.5	*	M	B
Y	7.4	20.8	42	M	B
N	5.2	27.9	56	M	B
Y	7.3	24.7	35	M	B
N	7.3	23.1	44	M	O
N	8.8	28.5	39	M	O
N	8.0	27.9	32	M	O
Y	5.3	25.5	37	M	O
N	5.2	26.0	22	M	O
N	5.1	22.4	24	M	O
N	5.4	24.6	31	M	O
N	6.5	28.7	36	M	O
N	6.0	28.5	43	M	O
N	6.6	28.7	47	M	O
Y	7.8	24.4	45	M	O
N	4.5	21.5	24	M	O
N	6.0	24.5	25	M	AB
Y	5.7	25.2	40	M	AB
N	4.6	23.0	23	M	AB
N	4.9	25.6	42	M	AB
N	5.9	27.3	20	M	AB
N	7.1	28.0	23	M	AB
N	5.9	31.7	24	M	AB
N	6.3	33.8	49	M	AB
N	6.3	27.6	27	M	AB
N	3.4	22.5	43	M	AB
N	4.7	25.2	36	M	B
N	8.7	28.8	30	F	B
N	5.2	25.7	43	F	B
N	6.8	26.3	47	M	B
Y	7.4	31.2	28	F	B

Table G.1. (cont.)

Smoke	wbc	bmi	Age	Sex	Blood group
Y	6.8	20.9	32	F	O
Y	10.6	28.0	42	F	B
Y	8.3	22.6	29	F	A
N	4.4	26.5	24	F	A
Y	9.6	21.1	21	M	B
Y	6.9	20.2	40	F	A

Table G.2. *Descriptive statistics for the three continuous predictors (wbc; white blood cell count; bmi, body mass index; age). The means are given with the standard errors in parentheses. Also shown are the results of unpaired t-tests, whose p-values have not been corrected for multiple testing*

	n	wbc	bmi	Age
Smoke	66	6.06 (0.18)	26.93 (0.46)	33.52 (1.09)
Non-smoke	21	7.26 (0.36)	25.14 (0.76)	34.76 (1.57)
t		−2.99	2.03	−0.65
p		0.01	0.05	0.52

References

AI Repository (1997). Genetic algorithms FAQ. Available online at
http://www.cs.cmu.edu/Groups/AI/html/faqs/ai/genetic/top.html (accessed
20 January 2006).

Allen, J.E., Pertea, M. and Salzberg, S.L. (2004). Computational gene prediction using
multiple sources of evidence. *Genome Research*, **14**, 142–8.

Altinçay, H. and Demirekler, M. (2003). Undesirable effects of output
normalization in multiple classifier systems. *Pattern Recognition Letters*, **24**,
1163–70.

Altman, D.G. and Bland, M.J. (1994). Statistics notes. Diagnostic tests
1: sensitivity and specificity. *British Medical Journal*, **308**, 1552. Available online
at http://bmj.bmjjournals.com/cgi/content/full/308/6943/1552 (accessed
24 October 2005).

Altman, D.G. and Royston, P. (2000). What do we mean by validating a prognostic
model? *Statistics in Medicine*, **19**(4), 453–73.

Andrews, R.L. and Melton, K.I. (1987). Incorporating misclassification costs into
computer package discriminant procedures. *Proceedings of the Southeast Chapter of
the Institute of Management Science*, **XVII**, 362–3.

Apostol, I. and Szpankowski, W. (1999). Indexing and mapping of proteins using a
modified nonlinear Sammon projection. *Journal of Computational Chemistry*, **20**(10),
1049–59.

Armengol, E. and Plaza, E. (2003). Relational case-based reasoning for carcinogenic
activity prediction. *Artificial Intelligence Review*, **20**, 121–41.

Aronow, B.J., Richardson, B.D. and Handwerger, S. (2001). Microarray analysis of
trophoblast differentiation: gene expression reprogramming in key gene
function categories. *Physiological Genomics*, **6**, 105–16.

Azuaje, F., Wang, H. and Chesneau, A. (2005). Non-linear mapping for exploratory
data analysis in functional genomics. *BMC Bioinformatics*, **6**, 13.
The electronic (complete) version of this article can be found online at
http://www.biomedcentral.com/1471-2105/6/13 (accessed 7 October 2005).

Baldi, P., Brunak, S., Chauvin, Y., Andersen, C.A.F. and Nielsen, H. (2000). Assessing the accuracy of prediction algorithms for classification: an overview. *Bioinformatics*, **16**(5), 412–24.

Bauer, E. and Kohavi, R. (1999). An empirical comparison of voting classification algorithms: bagging, boosting and variants. *Machine Learning*, **36**, 105–39.

Bell, J.F. (1999). Tree based methods. In A.H. Fielding, ed., *Machine Learning Methods for Ecological Applications*. Boston, MA: Kluwer Academic, pp. 89–106.

Ben-Hur, A. and Guyon, I. (2003). Detecting stable clusters using principal component analysis. In M.J. Brownstein and A. Khodursky, eds., *Methods in Molecular Biology*. Totowa, N J: Humana Press, pp. 159–82.

Bertin, J. (Berg, W.J., translation from French) (1967. Reprint 1983). *Semiology of Graphics: Diagrams, Networks and Maps*. Madison, WI: University of Wisconsin Press.

Bickel, D.R. (2003). Robust cluster analysis of microarray gene expression data with the number of clusters determined biologically. *Bioinformatics*, **19**(7), 818–24.

Bland, M.J. and Altman, D.G. (2000). Statistics notes: the odds-ratio. *British Medical Journal*, **320**, 1468. Available online at http://bmj.bmjjournals.com/cgi/content/full/320/7247/1468 (accessed 24 October 2005).

Blayo, F., Chevenal, Y., Guérin-Dugué, A., Chentouf, R., Aviles-Cruz, C., Madrenas, J., Moreno, M. and Voz, J.L. (1995). *Enhanced Learning for Evolutive Neural Architecture. Deliverable R3-B4-P Task B4: Benchmarks*. ESPIRIT Basic Research Project Number 6891.

Bo, H.Y. (2000). Knowledge discovery and data mining techniques and practice. Available at http://www.netnam.vn/unescocourse/knowlegde/knowlegd.htm and also in Word format from the same page (accessed 10 January 2006).

Bo, T. and Jonassen, I. (2002). New feature subset selection procedures for classification of expression profiles. *Genome Biology*, **3**, research0017.1–0017.11. Available online at http://genomebiology.com/2002/3/4/research/0017 (accessed 8 January 2006).

Boddy, L. and Morris, C.W. (1999). Artificial neural networks for pattern recognition. In A.H. Fielding, ed., *Ecological Applications of Machine Learning Methods*. Boston, MA: Kluwer Academic, pp. 37–69.

Boddy, L., Morris, C.W., Wilkins, M.F., Al-Haddad, L., Tarran, G.A., Jonker, R.R. and Burkill, P.H. (2000). Identification of 72 phytoplankton species by radial basis function neural network analysis of flow cytometric data. *Marine Ecology-Progress Series*, **195**, 47–59.

Bonnet, E. and Van de Peer, Y. (2002). zt: a software tool for simple and partial Mantel tests. *Journal of Statistical Software*, **7**(10), 1–12. Available online at http://www.jstatsoft.org/index.php?vol=7 (accessed 4 November 2005).

Breiman, L. (1996). Bagging predictors. *Machine Learning*, **24**, 123–40.

Breiman, L. (2001a). Random forests. *Machine Learning*, **45**, 5–32.

Breiman, L. (2001b). Statistical modelling: the two cultures. *Statistical Science*, **16**, 199–215.

Breiman, L. (2002). Manual on setting up, using, and understanding Random Forests V3.1. Available at http://oz.berkeley.edu/users/breiman/Using_random_forests_V3.1.pdf (accessed 2 February 2006).

Breiman, L. and Cutler, A. (2004a). Interface Workshop: April 2004. Available at http://
stat-www.berkeley.edu/users/breiman/RandomForests/interface04.pdf
(accessed 1 February 2006).

Breiman, L. and Cutler, A. (2004b). Random Forests. Available at
http://stat-www.berkeley.edu/users/breiman/RandomForests/cc_home.htm
(accessed 1 February 2006).

Breiman, L., Friedman, J.H., Olshen, R.A. and Stone, C.J. (1984). *Classification and
Regression Trees*. Monterey, CA: Wadsworth and Brooks.

Brillinger, D.R. (2002). John W. Tukey: his life and professional contributions.
The Annals of Statistics, **30**(6), 1535–75.

Brosse, S. and Lek, S. (2000). Modelling roach (*Rutilus rutilus*) microhabitat using linear
and nonlinear techniques. *Freshwater Biology*, **44**, 441–52.

Brown, M.P.S., Grundy, W.N., Lin, D., Cristianini, N., Sugnet, C.W., Furey, T.S.,
Ares, Jr., M. and Haussler, D. (2000). Knowledge-based analysis of microarray
gene expression data by using support vector machines. *Proceedings of the
National Academy of Sciences*, **97**(1), 262–67. Available as a pdf file at
http://www.pnas.org/cgi/reprint/97/1/262 (accessed 11 January 2006).

Bryan, J. (2004). Problems in gene clustering based on gene expression data. *Journal of
Multivariate Analysis*, **90**, 44–60.

Burbidge, R., Trotter, M., Buxton, B. and Holden, S. (1998). Drug design by machine
learning: support vector machines for pharmaceutical data analysis. *Computers
and Chemistry*, **26**, 5–14.

Burges, C.J.C. (1998). A tutorial on support vector machines for pattern recognition.
Data Mining and Knowledge Discovery, **2**(2), 1–47.

Burnham, K.P. and Anderson, D.R. (2002). *Model Selection and Multimodel Inference:
A Practical Information-Theoretic Approach*, 2nd edn. New York: Springer-Verlag.

Burnham, K.P. and Anderson, D.R. (2004). Multimodel inference: understanding
AIC and BIC in model selection. Amsterdam Workshop on Model Selection.
Available online at http://www2.fmg.uva.nl/modelselection/presentations/
AWMS2004-Burnham-paper.pdf (accessed 8 January 2006).

Calinski, R.B. and Harabasz, J. (1974). A dendrite method for cluster analysis.
Communication in Statistics, **3**, 1–27.

Carbonell, J.G. (1990). Introduction: paradigms for machine learning.
In J.G. Carbonell, ed., *Machine Learning: Paradigms and Methods*. Cambridge,
MA: MIT/Elsevier, pp. 1–10.

Castresana, J., Guigo, R. and Alba, M.M. (2004). Clustering of genes coding for DNA
binding proteins in a region of atypical evolution of the human genome.
Journal of Molecular Evolution, **59**(1), 72–9.

Chang, C.L. and Lee, R.C.T. (1973). A heuristic relaxation method for nonlinear
mapping in cluster analysis. *IEEE Transactions on Systems, Man, and Cybernetics*,
3, 197–200.

Chatfield, C. (1995). Model uncertainty, data mining and statistical
inference. *Journal of the Royal Statistical Society Series A, Statistics in Society*, **158**,
419–66.

Cheeseman, P. and Stutz, J. (1996). Bayesian classification (AutoClass): theory and results. In U.M. Fayyad, G. Piatetsky-Shapiro, P. Smyth and R. Uthurusamy, eds., *Advances in Knowledge Discovery and Data Mining*. AAAI Press/MIT Press, pp. 61–83. Available as a postscript file at http://ic.arc.nasa.gov/ic/projects/bayes-group/images/kdd-95.ps.

Chen, C.H. (2002). Generalized association plots: information visualization via iteratively generated correlation matrices. *Statistica Sinica*, **12**, 7–29. Available online at http://gap.stat.sinica.edu.tw/Papers/GAP_2002.pdf (accessed 8 October 2005).

Chen, C.H. and Chen, J.A. (2000). Interactive diagnostic plots for multidimensional scaling with applications in psychosis disorder data analysis. *Statistica Sinica*, **10**, 665–91.

Cheng, B. and Titterington, D.M. (1994). Neural networks: a review from a statistical perspective. *Statistical Science*, **9**, 2–54.

Chevan, A. and Sutherland, M. (1991). Hierarchical partitioning. *American Statistician*, **45**(2), 90–6.

Chipman, H. and Tibshirani, R. (2005). Hybrid hierarchical clustering with applications to microarray data. *Biostatistics*, online publication doi:10.1093/biostatistics/kxj007. Also available as a technical report in pdf format at http://www-stat.stanford.edu/~tibs/ftp/chipman-tibshirani-2003-modified.pdf (accessed 15 January 2006).

Clarke, R.T., Rothery, P. and Raybould, A.F. (2002). Confidence limits for regression relationships between distance matrices: estimating gene flow with distance. *Journal of Agricultural, Biological and Environmental Statistics*, **7**, 361–72. DISTMAT can be downloaded from http://www.ceh.ac.uk/products/software/CEHSoftware-Genetics-DISTMAT.html (accessed 12 October 2005).

Conroy, M.J., Cohen, Y., James, F.C., Matsinos, Y.G. and Maurer, B.A. (1995). Parameter estimation, reliability, and model improvement for spatially explicit models of animal populations. *Ecological Applications*, **5**, 17–9.

Cox, D.R. and Snell, E.J. (1989). *The Analysis of Binary Data*, 2nd edn. London: Chapman and Hall.

Cummings, M.P. and Myers, D.S. (2004). Simple statistical models predict C-to-U edited sites in plant mitochondria RNA. *BMC Bioinformatics*, **5**, 132. Available at http://www.biomedcentral.com/1471-2105/5/132 (accessed 2 February 2006).

Davis, E.B. (2005). Comparison of climate space and phylogeny of Marmota (Mammalia: Rodentia) indicates a connection between evolutionary history and climate preference. *Proceedings of the Royal Society B: Biological Sciences*, **272**(1562), 519–26.

Davis, J.C. (1986). *Statistics and Data Analysis in Geology*. London: John Wiley & Sons.

Deb, K. and Reddy, A.R. (2003). Reliable classification of two-class cancer data using evolutionary algorithms. *Biosystems*, **72**, 111–29.

Deleo, J.M. (1993). Receiver operating characteristic laboratory (ROCLAB): software for developing decision strategies that account for uncertainty. In *Proceedings of the*

Second International Symposium on Uncertainty Modelling and Analysis. College Park, MD: IEEE, Computer Society Press, pp. 318–25.

Deleo, J. M. and Campbell, G. (1990). The fuzzy receiver operating characteristic function and medical decisions with uncertainty. In *Proceedings of the First International Symposium on Uncertainty Modelling and Analysis*. College Park, MD: IEEE, Computer Society Press.

Dettling, M. (2004). BagBoosting for tumour classification with gene expression data. *Bioinformatics*, **20**(18), 3583–93. Available online at http://bioinformatics. oxfordjournals.org/cgi/screenpdf/20/18/3583.pdf (accessed 10 January 2006).

Dettling, M. and Bühlmann, P. (2004). Finding predictive gene groups from microarray data. *Journal of Multivariate Analysis*, **90**, 106–31.

Do, M. T., Harp, J. M. and Norris, K. C. (1999). A test of a pattern recognition system for identification of spiders. *Bulletin of Entomological Research*, **89**, 217–24.

Domingos, P. (1999). The role of Occam's Razor in knowledge discovery. *Data Mining and Knowledge Discovery*, **3**, 409–25.

Dougherty, E. R. (2001). Small sample issues for microarray-based classification. *Comparative and Functional Genomics*, **2**, 28–34.

Duda, R. O., Hart, P. E. and Stork, D. G. (2001). *Pattern Classification*, 2nd edn. New York: John Wiley & Sons.

Dudoit, S. and Fridlyand, J. (2003). Classification in microarray experiments. In T. P. Speed, ed., *Statistical Analysis of Gene Expression Microarray Data*. Chapman and Hall/CRC, pp. 93–158.

Dudoit, S., Fridlyand, J. and Speed, T. P. (2002). Comparison of discrimination methods for the classification of tumours using gene expression data. *Journal of the American Statistical Association*, **97**(457), 77–87.

Duin, R. P. W. (1996). A note on comparing classifiers. *Pattern Recognition Letters*, **17**, 529–36.

Dutton, D. M. and Conroy, G. V. (1996). A review of machine learning. *Knowledge Engineering Review*, **12**, 341–67.

Efron, B. and Tibshirani, R. J. (1993). *An Introduction to the Bootstrap*. London: Chapman and Hall.

Efron, B. and Tibshirani, R. (1997). Improvements on cross-validation: the 632+ bootstrap method. *Journal of the American Statistical Association*, **92**, 548–60.

Eisen, M. B., Spellman, P. T., Browndagger, P. O. and Botstein, D. (1998). Cluster analysis and display of genome-wide expression patterns. *Proceedings National Academy of Science USA*, **95**(25), 14863–8. Available at http://www.pnas.org/cgi/reprint/95/25/14863 (accessed 3 October 2005).

Estivill-Castro, V. and Yang, J. (2004). Fast and robust general purpose clustering algorithms. *Data Mining and Knowledge Discovery*, **28**, 127–50.

Everitt, B., Landau, S. and Leese, M. (2001). *Cluster Analysis*, 4th edn. Arnold, London.

Fawcett, T. (2003). *ROC Graphs: Notes and Practical Considerations for Data Mining Researchers*. Available for download from www.hpl.hp.com/techreports/2003/HPL-2003–4.pdf (6 October 2005).

Fielding, A. H. (1999a). A review of machine learning methods. In A. H. Fielding, ed., *Ecological Applications of Machine Learning Methods*. Boston, MA: Kluwer Academic, pp. 1–37.

Fielding, A. H. (1999b). How should accuracy be measured? In A. H. Fielding, ed., *Ecological Applications of Machine Learning Methods*. Boston, MA: Kluwer Academic, pp. 209–23.

Fielding, A. H. (2002). What are the appropriate characteristics of an accuracy measure? In J. M. Scott, P. J. Heglund, M. Morrison, J. B. Haufler, M. G. Raphael, W. B. Wall and F. Samson, eds., *Predicting Plant and Animal Occurrences: Issues of Scale and Accuracy*. Island Press, pp. 271–80.

Fielding, A. H. and Bell, J. F. (1997). A review of methods for the assessment of prediction errors in conservation presence/absence models. *Environmental Conservation*, **24**, 38–49.

Fielding, A. H. and Haworth, P. F. (1995). Testing the generality of bird-habitat models. *Conservation Biology*, **9**, 1466–81.

Filho, J. L. R., Treleavan, P. C. and Alippi, C. (1994). Genetic-algorithm programming environments. *Computer*, June, 29–43.

Filliben, J. J. and Heckert, A. (2002). DATAPLOT: multi-platform (Unix, VMS, Linux, Windows 95/98/ME/XP/NT/2000, etc.) software system for scientific visualization, statistical analysis, and non-linear modeling. Statistical Engineering Division, Information Technology Laboratory, National Institute of Standards and Technology. Available online at http://www.itl.nist.gov/div898/software/dataplot/ (accessed 5 October 2005).

Flexer, A. (1996). Statistical evaluation of neural network experiments: minimum requirements and current practice. In R. Trappl, ed., *Cybernetics and Systems '96: Proceedings of the 13th European Meeting on Cybernetics and Systems Research*. Austrian Society for Cybernetic Studies, pp. 1005–8.

Fodor, I. K. (2002). A survey of dimension reduction techniques. US Department of Energy. Available at http://www.llnl.gov/tid/lof/documents/pdf/240921.pdf (accessed 2 December 2005).

Forbes, A. D. (1995). Classification algorithm evaluation: five performance measures based on confusion matrices. *Journal of Clinical Monitoring*, **11**, 189–206.

Forman, G. (2002). A method for discovering the insignificance of one's best classifier and the unlearnability of a classification task. In Lavrac *et al.*, eds., *Proceedings of First International Workshop on Data Mining Lessons Learned (DMLL-2002)*. Available at http://www.hpl.hp.com/techreports/2002/HPL-2002-123R2.pdf (accessed 6 October 2005).

Forsyth, R. (1981). BEAGLE: a Darwinian approach to pattern recognition. *Kybernetes*, **10**(3), 159–66.

Fox, A. D., Jones, T. A., Singleton, R. and Agnew, A. D. Q. (1994). Food supply and the effects of recreational disturbance on the abundance and distribution of wintering pochard on a gravel pit complex in southern Britain. *Hydrobiologia*, **279/280**, 253–61.

Freund, Y. and Schapire, R. E. (1996). Experiments with a new boosting algorithm. In *Machine Learning: Proceedings of the Thirteenth International Conference*. San Francisco, CA: Morgan Kauffman, pp. 148−56.

Friedman, J. H. (1997). On bias, variance, 0/1 − loss and the curse of dimensionality. *Data Mining and Knowledge Discovery*, **1**, 55−77.

Friedman, J. H., Hastie, T. and Tibshirani, R. (2000). Additive logistic regression: a statistical view of boosting. *Annals of Statistics*, **28**(2), 337−74.

Friendly, M. (2002). Corrgrams: exploratory displays for correlation matrices. *American Statistician*, **56**(4), 316−24.

Furey, T. S., Cristianini, N., Duffy, N., Bednarski, D. W., Schummer, M. and Haussler, D. (2000). Support vector machine classification and validation of cancer tissue samples using microarray expression data. *Bioinformatics*, **16**(10), 906−14. Available as a pdf file at http://bioinformatics.oxfordjournals.org/cgi/reprint/16/10/906 (accessed 20 January 2006).

Gaston, K. J. and O'Neill, M. A. (2004). Automated species identification: why not? *Philosophical Transactions of the Royal Society of London B*, **359**, 655−67. Available online at http://darwin.zoology.gla.ac.uk/~vsmith/conference/barcoding/download/Gaston_Neil.pdf (accessed 5 October 2005).

Gentleman, R. C., Carey, V. J., Bates, D. M., *et al.* (2004). Bioconductor: open software development for computational biology and bioinformatics. *Genome Biology*, **5**, R80. Available at http://genomebiology.com/2004/5/10/R80 (accessed 10 January 2006).

Geverey, M., Dimopoulos, I. and Lek, S. (2003). Review and comparison of methods to study the contribution of variables in artificial neural network models. *Ecological Modelling*, **160**, 249−64.

Gilbert, E. D. (1969). The effect of unequal variance covariance matrices on Fisher's linear discriminant function. *Biometrics*, **25**, 505−15.

Giraud-Carrier, C. G. and Martinez, T. R. (1995). An integrated framework for learning and reasoning. *Journal of Artificial Intelligence Research*, **3**, 147−85.

Golub, T. R., Slonim, D. K., Tamayo, P., Huard, C., Gaasenbeek, M., Mesirov, J. P., Coller, H., Loh, M., Downing, J. R., Caligiuri, M. A., Bloomfield, C. D. and Lander, E. S. (1999). Molecular classification of cancer: class discovery and class prediction by gene expression. *Science*, **286**, 531−6. Available as a pdf file, plus associated data files at http://www.broad.mit.edu/cgi-bin/cancer/publications/pub_paper.cgi?mode=view&paper_id=43 (accessed 15 October 2005).

Goodman, P. H. (1996). *NevProp software, version 3*. Reno, NV: University of Nevada. Available at http://www.scs.unr.edu/nevprop/ (accessed 3 February 2006).

Goodman, P. H. and Harrell, F. E. (2001a). Neural networks: advantages and limitations for biostatistical modeling. Available at http://brain.cs.unr.edu/publications/goodman.ann_advantages.jasa99.pdf (accessed 3 February 2006).

Goodman, P. H. and Harrell, F. E. (2001b). *NevProp Manual with Introduction to Artificial Neural Network Theory*. Available at http://brain.cs.unr.edu/publications/NevPropManual.pdf (accessed 3 February 2006).

Goodman, P. H. and Rosen, D. B. (2001). *NevProp Artificial Neural Network Software with Cross-Validation and Bootstrapped Confidence Intervals*. Available at http://brain.cs.unr.edu/FILES_PHP/show_papers.php (accessed 20 January 2006).

Gordon, A. D. (1981). *Classification Methods for the Exploratory Analysis of Multivariate Data*. London: Chapman and Hall.

Gordon, A. D. (1999). *Classification*. London: Chapman and Hall.

Gower, J. (1971). A general coefficient of similarity and some of its properties. *Biometrics*, **27**, 857–74.

Grabmeier, J. and Rudolph, A. (2002). Techniques of cluster algorithms in data mining. *Data Mining and Knowledge Discovery*, **6**, 303–60.

Gregory, T. R. (2005). *Animal Genome Size Database*. Available at http://www.genomesize.com (accessed 7 January 2006).

Hall, P. and Samworth, R. J. (2005). Properties of bagged nearest neighbour classifiers. *Journal of the Royal Statistical Society, Series B*, **67**(3), 363–79.

Hammer, Ø., Harper, D. A. T. and Ryan, P. D. (2001). PAST: paleontological statistics software package for education and data analysis. *Palaeontologia Electronica*, **4**(1), 9pp. Available at http://palaeo-electronica.org/2001_1/past/issue1_01.htm (accessed 11 October 2005).

Hand, D. J. (1997). *Construction and Assessment of Classification Rules*. Chichester, UK: Wiley and Sons.

Hand, D. J. and Henley, W. E. (1997). Statistical classification methods in consumer credit scoring: a review. *Journal of the Royal Statistical Society, Series A*, **160**, 523–41.

Hastie, T. J. (1992). Generalized additive models. In J. M. Chambers and T. J. Hastie, eds., *Statistical Models in S*. Wadsworth and Brooks/Cole.

Hastie, T. J. and Tibshirani, R. J. (1990). *Generalized Additive Models*. London: Chapman and Hall.

Hastie, T. J. and Tibshirani, R. J. (1996). Discriminant analysis by Gaussian mixtures. *Journal of the Royal Statistical Society, Series B*, **58**, 155–76.

Hastie, T. J., Buja, A. and Tibshirani, R. J. (1995). Penalized discriminant analysis. *Annals of Statistics*, **23**, 73–102.

Hastie, T. J., Tibshirani, R. J. and Buja, A. (1994). Flexible discriminant analysis by optimal scoring. *Journal of the American Statistical Association*, **89**, 1255–70.

Hastie, T., Tibshirani, R., Eisen, M. B., Alizadeh, A., Levy, R., Staudt, L., Chan, W. C., Botstein, D. and Brown, P. (2000). 'Gene shaving' as a method for identifying distinct sets of genes with similar expression patterns. *Genome Biology*, **1**(2), research0003.1–0003.21. Available online at http://genomebiology.com/2000/1/2/research/0003.

Hauck, W. W. and Donner, A. (1977). Wald's test as applied to hypotheses in logit analysis. *Journal of the American Statistical Association*, **72**, 851–53.

Helsel, D. R. and Hirsch, R. M. (2005). *Statistical Methods in Water Resources. Techniques of Water-Resources Investigations of the United States Geological Survey Book 4, Hydrologic Analysis and Interpretation*. USGS. Available for download in pdf format at http://water.usgs.gov/pubs/twri/twri4a3/html/pdf_new.html (accessed 7 October 2005).

Henery, R. J. (1994). Classification. In D. Michie, D. J. Spiegelhalter and C. C. Taylor, eds., *Machine Learning, Neural and Statistical Classification*. New York: Ellis Horwood. pp. 6–16. Also available in a free, pdf format at http://www.maths.leeds.ac.uk/ %7Echarles/statlog/ (accessed 6 October 2005).

Heyer, L. J., Kruglyak, S. and Yooseph, S. (1999). Exploring expression data: identification and analysis of co-expressed genes. *Genome Research*, **9**, 1106–15.

Hill, M. O. (1979). TWINSPAN. *A FORTRAN Program for Arranging Multivariate Data in an Ordered Two-way Table by Classification of the Individuals and Attributes*. Ithaca, NY: Cornell University.

Hill, M. O. and Gauch, Jr, H. G. (1980). Detrended correspondence analysis: an improved ordination technique. *Vegetatio*, **42**, 47–58.

Hill, M. O. and Šmilauer, P. (2005). *TWINSPAN for Windows version 2.3*. Centre for Ecology and Hydrology & University of South Bohemia, Huntingdon & České Budějovice. Available at http://www.ceh.ac.uk/products/software/wintwins.html (accessed 12 October 2005).

Hollmen, J., Skubacz, M. and Taniguchi, M. (2000). Input dependent misclassification costs for cost-sensitive classifiers. In N. Ebecken and C. Brebbia, eds., *Proceedings of the Second International Conference on Data Mining*. Southampton: WIT Press, pp. 495–503. Available online at http://lib.tkk.fi/Diss/2000/isbn9512252392/ article5.pdf (accessed 30 October 2005).

Hood, G. (2005). *Poptools Version 2.6 (build 9)*. Released 1 October 2005. Available at http://www.cse.csiro.au/poptools/index.htm (accessed 7 October 2005).

Hosking, J. R. M., Pednault, E. P. D. and Sudan, M. (1997). A statistical perspective on data mining. *Future Generation Computer Systems*, **13**, 117–34.

Hosmer, D. W. and Lemeshow, S. (1989). *Applied Logistic Regression*. New York: Wiley.

Huberty, C. J. (1994). *Applied Discriminant Analysis*. New York: Wiley Interscience.

Intrator, O. and Intrator, N. (2001). Interpreting neural-network results: a simulation study. *Computational Statistics and Data Analysis*, **37**(3), 373–93.

Jain, A. K., Dubes, R. C. and Chen, C.-C. (1987). Bootstrap techniques for error estimation. *IEEE Transactions on Pattern Analysis and Machine Intelligence*, **9**(5), 628–33.

Jain, A. K., Duin, R. P. W. and Mao, J. (2000). Statistical pattern recognition: a review. *IEEE Transactions on Pattern Analysis and Machine Intelligence*, **22**(1), 4–37.

Jain, A. K., Topchy, A., Law, M. H. C. and Buhmann, J. M. (2004). Landscape of clustering algorithms. *Proceedings of the 17th International Conference on Pattern Recognition*, **1**, 260–3.

Jeffers, J. N. R. (1996). Multivariate analysis of a reference collection of elm leaves. *Journal of Applied Statistics*, **23**, 571–87.

Jeffers, J. N. R. (1999). Genetic algorithms I. Ecological applications of the BEAGLE and GAFFER genetic algorithms. In A. Fielding, ed., *Ecological Applications of Machine Learning Methods*. Boston, MA: Kluwer Academic, pp. 107–15.

Jenkins, J. A. (1991). A study of machine variables and donor characteristics: their effect on the quality of plasma obtained from haemonetics PCS plasmapheresis. Unpublished M.Sc. thesis, Manchester Metropolitan University.

Jirapech-Umpai, T. and Aitken, S. (2005). Feature selection and classification for microarray data analysis: evolutionary methods for identifying predictive genes. *BMC Bioinformatics*, **6**, 148. Available at http://www.biomedcentral.com/1471–2105/6/148.

Jongman, R. H. G., ter Braak, C. F. R. and van Tongeren, O. F. R. (1995). *Data Analysis in Community and Landscape Ecology*. Cambridge: Cambridge University Press.

Kannel, W. B., Anderson, K. and Wilson, P. W. (1992). White blood cell count and cardiovascular disease. Insights from the Framingham Study. *JAMA*, **267**(9), 1253–6.

Karzynski, M., Mateos, Á., Herrero, J. and Dopazo, J. (2003). Using a genetic algorithm and a perceptron for feature selection and supervised class learning in DNA microarray studies. *Artificial Intelligence Review*, **20**, 39–51.

Kass, G. V. (1980). An exploratory technique for investigating large quantities of categorical data. *Applied Statistics*, **29**, 119–27.

Kaufman, L. and Rousseeuw, P. J. (1990). *Finding Groups in Data: An Introduction to Cluster Analysis*. Wiley.

Kaufman, L. and Rousseeuw, P. J. (2005). *Finding Groups in Data. An Introduction to Cluster Analysis*. New Jersey: Wiley-Interscience.

Kohavi, R. (1995). A study of cross-validation and bootstrap for accuracy estimation and model selection. In C. S. Mellish, ed., *Proceedings of the 14th International Joint Conference on Artificial Intelligence*. San Francisco, CA: Morgan Kaufmann, pp. 1137–43. Available at http://robotics.stanford.edu/~ronnyk (accessed 24 October 2005).

Kohonen, T. (1988). An introduction to neural computing. *Neural Networks*, **1**, 3–16.

Kohonen, T. (1990). The self-organising map. *Proceedings of IEEE*, **78**, 1464–80.

Lance, G. N. and Williams, W. T. (1967). A general theory of classificatory sorting strategies. *Computer Journal*, **9**, 373–80.

Landis, J. R. and Koch, G. C. (1977). The measurement of observer agreement for categorical data. *Biometrics*, **33**, 159–74.

Lapointe, F. J. and Legendre, P. (1994). A classification of pure malt Scotch whiskies. *Applied Statistics*, **43**(1), 237–57. Also available in a modified form at http://www.dcs.ed.ac.uk/home/jhb/whisky/lapointe/text.html (accessed 2 October 2005).

Lee, J. W., Lee, J. B., Park, M. and Songa, S. H. (2005). An extensive comparison of recent classification tools applied to microarray data. *Computational Statistics and Data Analysis*, **48**, 869–85.

Legendre, P. and Lapointe, F.-J. (2004). Assessing congruence among distance matrices: single-malt Scotch whiskies revisited. *Australian and New Zealand Journal of Statistics*, **46**(4), 615–29.

Legendre, P. and Legendre, L. (1998). *Numerical Ecology*, 2nd English edn. Amsterdam: Elsevier.

Li, J., Liu, H., Ng, S.-K. and Wong, L. (2003). Discovery of significant rules for classifying cancer diagnosis data. *Bioinformatics*, **19** (Suppl. 2), i93–i102.

Liaw, A. and Wiener, A. (2006). *The randomForest package*. Available at http://cran.r-project.org/doc/packages/randomForest.pdf (accessed 3 February 2006).

Lim, T.-S., Loh, W.-H. and Shih, Y.-S. (2000). A comparison of prediction accuracy, complexity, and training time of thirty three old and new classification algorithms. *Machine Learning*, **40**, 203–29.

Lin, T. C. and Pourhmadi, M. (1998). Nonparametric and non-linear models and data mining in time series: a case study on the Canadian lynx data. *Applied Statistics*, **47**, 187–201.

Lingras, P. and Huang, X. (2005). Statistical, evolutionary and neurocomputing clustering techniques: cluster-based vs object-based approaches. *Artificial Intelligence Review*, **23**, 3–29.

Liu, J. J., Cutler, G., Li, W., Pan, Z., Peng, S., Hoey, T., Chen, L. and Ling, X. B. (2005). Multiclass cancer classification and biomarker discovery using GA-based algorithms. *Bioinformatics*, **21**, 2691–7.

Liu, X. H. (1996). Intelligent data analysis: issues and concepts. *Knowledge Engineering Review*, **11**, 365–7.

Loh, W. Y. and Shih, Y. S. (1997). Split selection methods for Classification trees. *Statistica Sinica*, **7**, 815–40.

Lynn, H., Mohler, C. L., DeGloria, S. D. and McCulloch, C. E. (1995). Error assessment in decision-tree models applied to vegetation analysis. *Landscape Ecology*, **10**, 323–35.

Ma, Z. and Redmond, R. L. (1995). Tau coefficients for accuracy assessment of classifications of remote sensing data. *Photogrammetric Engineering and Remote Sensing*, **61**, 435–9.

Mac Nally, R. (2000). Regression and model-building in conservation biology, biogeography and ecology: the distinction between – and reconciliation of – 'predictive' and 'explanatory' models. *Biodiversity and Conservation*, **9**, 655–71.

Madger, L. S. and Hughes, J. P. (1997). Logistic regression when the outcome is measured with uncertainty. *American Journal of Epidemiology*, **146**, 195–203.

Manel, S., Dias, J.-M. and Omerod, S. J. (1999a). Comparing discriminant analysis, neural networks and logistic regression for predicting species distributions: a case study with a Himalayan river bird. *Ecological Modelling*, **120**, 337–47.

Manel, S., Dias, J.-M., Buckton, S. and Omerod, S. J. (1999b). Alternative methods for predicting species distributions: an illustration with Himalayan river birds. *Journal of Applied Ecology*, **36**, 734–47.

Mangasarian, O. L. and Wolberg, W. H. (1990). Cancer diagnosis via linear programming. *SIAM News*, **23**(5), 1–18.

Mantel, N. (1967). The detection of disease clustering and a generalised regression approach. *Cancer Research*, **27**, 209–20.

Marks, S. and Dunn, O. J. (1974). Discriminant functions when covariance matrices are unequal. *Journal of the American Statistical Association*, **69**, 555–9.

Marsden, S. and Fielding, A. H. (1999). Habitat associations of parrots on the islands of Buru, Seram and Sumba. *Journal of Biogeography*, **26**, 439–46.

May, L. (1998). Individually distinctive corncrake *Crex crex* calls: a further study. *Bioacoustics*, **9**, 135–48.

McClelland, J.L., Rumelhart, D.E. and the PDP Research Group (eds.) (1986). *Parallel Distributed Processing*. Cambridge, MA: MIT Press.

Michie, D., Spiegelhalter, D.J. and Taylor, C.C. (eds.) (1994). *Machine Learning, Neural and Statistical Classification*. New York: Ellis Horwood. Also available in a free, pdf format at http://www.maths.leeds.ac.uk/%7Echarles/statlog/ (accessed 6 October 2005).

Milligan, G.W. and Cooper, M.C. (1985). An examination of procedures for determining the number of clusters in a data set. *Psychometrika*, **50**, 159–79.

Minsky, M. and Papert, S. (1969). *Perceptrons: An Introduction to Computational Geometry*. Cambridge, MA: MIT Press.

Murthy, S.K. (1998). Automatic construction of decision trees from data: a multi-disciplinary survey. *Data Mining and Knowledge Discovery*, **2**(4), 345–89.

Murthy, S.K., Kasif, S. and Salzberg, S. (1994). A system for induction of oblique decision trees. *Journal of Artificial Intelligence Research*, **2**, 1–32. Available as a pdf file at http://www.cs.cmu.edu/afs/cs/project/jair/pub/volume2/murthy94a.pdf (accessed 18 January 2006).

Myers, L., Riggs, M., Lashley, J. and Whitmore, R. (2000). *Options for Development of Parametric Probability Distributions for Exposure Factors*. Washington, DC: National Center for Environmental Assessment, Washington Office, Office of Research and Development, US Environmental Protection Agency. Available online at http://www.epa.gov/ncea/pdfs/paramprob4ef/finalTOC.pdf (accessed 8 October 2005).

Nagelkerke, N.J.D. (1991). A note on a general definition of the coefficient of determination. *Biometrika*, **78**(3), 691–2.

NIST/SEMATECH e-Handbook of Statistical Methods, Available at http://www.itl.nist.gov/div898/handbook/ (accessed 8 October 2005).

Olden, J.D., Joy, M.K. and Death, R.G. (2004). An accurate comparison of methods for quantifying variable importance in artificial neural networks using simulated data. *Ecological Modelling*, **178**, 389–97.

Perrière, G. and Thioulouse, J. (2002). Use and misuse of correspondence analysis in codon usage studies. *Nucleic Acids Research*, **30**(20), 4548–55.

Pillar, V.D. (1999). How sharp are classifications? *Ecology*, **80**, 2508–16.

Prasad, A.M., Iverson, L.R. and Liaw, A. (in press). Newer classification and regression tree techniques: bagging and Random Forests for ecological prediction. *Ecosystems*, **9**, 181–99.

Prechelt, L. (1997). A quantitative study of experimental evaluations of neural network algorithms: current research practice. *Neural Networks*, **9**, 317–27.

Proches, S. (2005). The world's biogeographic regions: cluster analysis based on bat distributions. *Journal of Biogeography*, **32**, 607–14.

Provost, F. and Fawcett, T. (1997). Analysis and visualisation of classifier performance: comparison under imprecise class and cost distributions. In *Proceedings of the Third*

International Conference on Knowledge Discovery and Data Mining. Menlo Park, CA: AAAI Press, pp. 43–8.

Quackenbush, J. (2001). Computational analysis of microarray data. *Nature Reviews Genetics*, **2**(6), 418–27.

Quinlan, J. (1983). Learning efficient classification procedures and their applications to chess end games. In R. Michalski, R. Carbonell and T. Mitchell, eds., *Machine Learning: An Artificial Intelligence Approach*, Vol. **1**. San Francisco, CA: Morgan Kaufmann, pp. 463–82.

Quinlan, R. J. (1979). Discovering rules from large collections of examples: a case study. In D. Michie, ed., *Expert Systems in the Micro-electronic Age*. Edinburgh: Edinburgh University Press, pp. 168–201.

Rataj, T. and Schlinder, J. (1991). Identification of bacteria by a multilayer neural network. *Binary*, **3**, 159–64.

Remaley, A. T., Sampson, M. L., DeLeo, J. M., Remaley, N. A., Farsi, B. D. and Zweig, M. H. (1999). Prevalence-value-accuracy plots: a new method for comparing diagnostic tests based on misclassification costs. *Clinical Chemistry*, **45**(7), 934–41. Available for download at http://www.clinchem.org/cgi/reprint/45/7/934.

Remm, K. (2004). Case-based predictions for species and habitat mapping. *Ecological Modelling*, **177**, 259–81.

Rencher, A. C. (1995). *Methods of Multivariate Analysis*. New York: Wiley.

Riordan, P. (1998). Unsupervised recognition of individual tigers and snow leopards from their footprints. *Animal Conservation*, **1**, 253–62.

Ripley, B. D. (1996). *Pattern Recognition and Neural Networks*. Cambridge: Cambridge University Press.

Rogers, S., Williams, R. D. and Campbell, C. (2005). Class prediction with microarray datasets. In U. Seiffert, L. C. Jain and P. Schweizer, eds., *Bioinformatics using Computational Intelligence Paradigms*. Springer, pp. 119–41.

Salzberg, S. L. (1997). On comparing classifiers: pitfalls to avoid and a recommended approach. *Data Mining and Knowledge Discovery*, **1**, 317–27.

Sammon, J. W. (1969). A nonlinear mapping for data structure analysis. *IEEE Transactions on Computers*, **C-18**(5), 401–9.

Sarle, W. S. (1994). Neural networks and statistical models. In *Proceedings of the Nineteenth Annual SAS Users Group International Conference*, Cary, NC: SAS Institute, pp. 1538–50. Available in postscript format from ftp://ftp.sas.com/pub/neural/neural1.ps.

Sasson, O., Linial, N. and Linial, M. (2002). The metric space of proteins: comparative study of clustering algorithms. *Bioinformatics*, **18**(Suppl. 1), S14–S21.

Schaafsma, W. and van Vark, G. N. (1979). Classification and discrimination problems with applications. Part IIa. *Statistica Neerlandica*, **33**, 91–126.

Schapire, R. E. (1990). The strength of weak learnability. *Machine Learning*, **5**(2), 197–227.

Schiffers, J. (1997). A classification approach incorporating misclassification costs. *Intelligent Data Analysis*, **1**, 59–68.

Schmelzer, I. (2000). Seals and seascapes: covariation in Hawaiian monk seal subpopulations and the oceanic landscape of the Hawaiian Archipelago. *Journal of Biogeography*, **27**, 901–14.

Schwarzer, G., Vach, W. and Schumacher, M. (2000). On the misuses of artificial neural networks for prognostic and diagnostic classification in oncology. *Statistics in Medicine*, **19**, 541–61.

Segal, M. R., Barbour, J. D. and Grant, R. M. (2004). Relating HIV-1 sequence variation to replication capacity via trees and forests. *Statistical Application in Genetics and Molecular Biology*, **3**(1), article 2. Available at http://www.bepress.com/sagmb/vol3/iss1/art2/ (accessed 3 February 2006).

Slonin, D. K. (2002). From patterns to pathways: gene expression data analysis comes of age. *Nature Genetics Supplement*, **32**, 502–8.

Sneath, P. H. and Sokal, R. R. (1973). *Numerical Taxonomy: The Principles and Practice of Numerical Classification*. San Francisco: Freeman.

South, M. C. (1994). The application of genetic algorithms to rule finding in data analysis. Unpublished Ph.D. thesis, University of Newcastle upon Tyne.

Spinks, P. Q. and Shaffer, H. B. (2005). Range-wide molecular analysis of the western pond turtle (*Emys marmorata*): cryptic variation, isolation by distance, and their conservation implications. *Molecular Ecology*, **14**(7), 2047–64.

Stafanescu, C., Penuelas, J. and Filella, I. (2005). Butterflies highlight the conservation value of hay meadows highly threatened by land-use changes in a protected Mediterranean area. *Biological Conservation*, **126**(2), 234–46.

Stephens, P. A., Buskirk, S. W., Hayward, G. D. and Martínez del Rio, C. (2005). Information theory and hypothesis testing: a call for pluralism. *Journal of Applied Ecology*, **42**, 4–12.

Stevens-Wood, B. (1999). Real learning. In A. H. Fielding, ed., *Ecological Applications of Machine Learning Methods*. Boston, MA: Kluwer Academic, pp. 225–46.

Stockwell, D. R. B. (1992). Machine learning and the problem of prediction and explanation in ecological modelling. Unpublished Ph.D. thesis, Australian National University.

Stockwell, D. R. B. (1993). LBS: Bayesian learning system for rapid expert system development. *Expert Systems with Applications*, **6**, 137–48.

Stockwell, D. R. B. (1999). Genetic algorithms II. In A. Fielding, ed., *Ecological Applications of Machine Learning Methods*. Boston, MA: Kluwer Academic, pp. 123–37.

Stockwell, D. R. B. and Noble, I. R. (1992). Induction of sets of rules from animal distribution data: a robust and informative method of data analysis. *Mathematics and Computers in Simulation*, **32**, 249–54.

Stockwell, D. R. B. and Peters, D. P. (1999). The GARP modelling system: problems and solutions to automated spatial prediction. *International Journal of Geographic Information Systems*, **13**, 143–58.

Swets, J. A., Dawes, R. and Monahan, J. (2000). Better decisions through science. *Scientific American*, October, 70–5.

ter Braak, C.J.F. (1986). Canonical correspondence analysis: a new eigenvector technique for multivariate direct gradient analysis. *Ecology*, **67**, 1167–79.

ter Braak, C.J.F. (1987). The analysis of vegetation–environment relationships by canonical correspondence analysis. *Vegetatio*, **69**, 69–77.

Tibshirani, R., Hastie, T., Eisen, M., Ross, D., Botstein, D. and Brown, P. (1999). *Clustering Methods for the Analysis of DNA Microarray Data*. Technical report, Department of Statistics, Stanford University. Available as a postscript file at http://www-stat.stanford.edu/~tibs/ftp/sjcgs.ps (accessed 17 January 2006).

Tibshirani, R., Walther, G. and Hastie, T. (2001). Estimating the number of clusters in a dataset via the Gap statistic. *Journal of the Royal Statistical Society, Series B*, **63**, 411–23. Also available as technical report from the Department of Statistics, Stanford University (pdf format) at http://www-stat.stanford.edu/~tibs/ftp/gap.pdf (accessed 10 January 2006).

Tufte, E.R. (1997). *Visual Explanations: Images and Quantities, Evidence and Narrative*. Reading, MA: Addison-Wesley.

Tukey, J.W. (1969). Analyzing data: sanctification or detective work? *American Psychologist*, **24**, 83–91.

Tukey, J.W. (1977). *Exploratory Data Analysis*. Reading, MA: Addison-Wesley.

Tukey, J.W. (1986). Sunset salvo. *American Statistician*, **40**, 72–6.

Turney, P.D. (1995). Cost-sensitive classification: empirical evaluation of a hybrid genetic decision tree induction algorithm. *Journal of Artificial Intelligence Research*, **2**, 369–409.

Turney, P.D. (2000). Types of cost in inductive concept learning. *Proceedings of the Cost-Sensitive Learning Workshop at the 17th ICML-2000 Conference*, Stanford, CA. Available online at http://www.cs.bilkent.edu.tr/~guvenir/courses/cs550/Seminar/NRC-43671.pdf (accessed 24 October 2005).

Upton, G. (1992). Fisher's exact test. *Journal of the Royal Statistical Society. Series A (Statistics in Society)*, **155**, 395–402.

Watanabe, S. (1985). *Pattern Recognition: Human and Mechanical*. New York: John Wiley & Sons.

Watson, I. and Marir, F. (1994). Case-based reasoning: A review. Available at http://www.ai-cbr.org/classroom/cbr-review.html (accessed 20 January 2006).

Wehrens, R., Putter, H. and Buydens, L.M.C. (2000). The bootstrap: a tutorial. *Chemometrics and Intelligent Laboratory Systems*, **54**, 35–52.

Wikipedia (2005). http://en.wikipedia.org/wiki/Pattern_recognition (accessed 20 September 2005).

Wilkins, M.F., Hardy, S.A., Boddy, L. and Morris, C.W. (2001). Comparison of five clustering algorithms to classify phytoplankton from flow cytometry data. *Cytometry*, **44**(3), 210–7.

Witten, I.H. and Frank, E. (2005). *Data Mining: Practical Machine Learning Tools and Techniques*, 2nd edn. San Francisco, CA: Morgan Kaufmann.

Wolpert, D.H. and Macready, W.G. (1995). *No Free Lunch Theorems for Search*, technical report SFI-TR-95-02-010, Santa Fe Institute. Available online at http://www.no-free-lunch.org/WoMa95.pdf (accessed 6 October 2005).

Wood, B. and Collard, M. (1999). The human genus. *Science*, **284**, 6571.

Wren, J.D., Johnson, D. and Gruenwald, L. (2005). Automating genomic data mining via a sequence-based matrix format and associative set. *BMC Bioinformatics*, **6**(Suppl. 2), S2 doi: 10.1186/147-2105-6-S2-S2. Available online at http://www.biomedcentral.com/1471-2105/6/s2/s2 (accessed 12 January 2006).

Wu, H.M. and Chen, C.H. (2006). GAP: a graphical environment for matrix visualization and information mining. To be submitted. Software homepage: http://gap.stat.sinica.edu.tw/Software/GAP (accessed 17 January 2006).

Xiong, M., Jin, L., Li, W. and Beerwinkle, E. (2000). Computational methods for gene expression-based tumour classification. *Biotechniques*, **29**, 1264–70.

Yeang, C.H., Ramaswamy, S., Tamayo, P., Mukherjee, S., Rifkin, R.M., Angelo, M., Reich, M., Lander, E., Mesirov, J. and Golub, T. (2001). Molecular classification of multiple tumour types. *Bioinformatics*, **17**(Suppl. 1), S316–S322.

Zou, K.H. (2002). Receiver operating characteristic (ROC) literature research. Available online at http://splweb.bwh.harvard.edu:8000/pages/ppl/zou/roc.html (accessed 25 October 2005).

Zweig, M.H. and Campbell, G. (1993). Receiver-operating characteristic (ROC) plots: a fundamental evaluation tool in clinical medicine. *Clinical Chemistry*, **39**, 561–77.

Index